CBS

Quick Text Revision Series
Important Text for Viva/MCQs

PHARMACOLOGY
For MBBS, BDS & Other Exams

SECOND EDITION

Edited by:

Dr. M.S. Bhatia
M.D., F.I.P., Dip. W.P.A., M.N.A.M.S.
Prof. & Head, Department of Psychiatry,
University College of Medical Sciences,
Dilshad Garden, Delhi - 110 095 (India)

Contributing Editor:

Dr. Nirmaljit Kaur
M.D.
Prof., Department of Microbiology,
Dr. R.M.L. Hospital,
New Delhi - 110 001 (India)

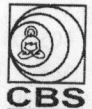

CBS

CBS Publishers & Distributors Pvt. Ltd.
New Delhi • Bengaluru • Chennai • Kochi • Kolkata • Mumbai
Hyderabad • Nagpur • Patna • Pune • Jharkhand • Uttarakhand

> **Dedicated to**
>
> **Respected Teachers & Beloved Students**

ISBN: 978-93-88902-79-3

First Edition: 2008
Reprint: 2009, 2014
Second Edition: 2019

Published by **Satish Kumar Jain** and produced by **Varun Jain** for
CBS Publishers & Distributors Pvt. Ltd.,
4819/XI Prahlad Street, 24 Ansari Road, Daryaganj, New Delhi - 110002
delhi@cbspd.com, cbspubs@airtelmail.in • www.cbspd.com
Ph.: 23289259, 23266861, 23266867 • Fax: 011-23243014

Corporate Office: 204 FIE, Industrial Area, Patparganj, Delhi - 110 092
Ph: 49344934 • Fax: 011-49344935
E-mail: publishing@cbspd.com • publicity@cbspd.com

Branches:
- *Bengaluru:* 2975, 17th Cross, K.R. Road, Bansankari 2nd Stage, Bengaluru - 70 • Ph: +91-80-26771678/79 • Fax: +91-80-26771680
  E-mail: cbsbng@gmail.com, bangalore@cbspd.com
- *Chennai:* No. 7, Subbaraya Street, Shenoy Nagar, Chennai - 600030
  Ph: +91-44-26681266, 26680620 • Fax: +91-44-42032115
  E-mail: chennai@cbspd.com
- *Kochi:* Ashana House, 39/1904, A.M. Thomas Road, Valanjambalam, Ernakulum, Kochi • Ph: +91-484-4059061-65
  Fax: +91-484-4059065 • E-mail: cochin@cbspd.com
- *Kolkata:* 6-B, Ground Floor, Rameshwar Shaw Road, Kolkata - 700014
  Ph: +91-33-22891126/7/8 • E-mail: kolkata@cbspd.com
- *Mumbai:* 83-C, Dr. E. Moses Road, Worli, Mumbai - 400018
  Ph: +91-9833017933, 022-24902340/41 • E-mail: mumbai@cbspd.com

Printed at: Neekunj Print Process, Delhi (India)

PREFACE

Medical science is a rapidly advancing field. Its new allied. branches are coming up. In a competitive examination, more and more emphasis is being laid on these allied disciplines. But most of the standard textbooks of medicine have failed to devote adequate space to these new disciplines.

This new Quick Text Revision Series has been written with the aim to outline the major areas of various subjects.

Pharmacology includes Factual Data, Important Points for Viva/MCQ's Important Text from General Pharmacology, CVS, CNS, Endocrinology Chemotherapy etc.

This book will also be useul for MBBS, BDS and Entrance Examinations

All suggestions for the modification of this book are welcome and will be duly acknowledged.

—Editors

Contents

Preface   iii

1. Factual Data   1–3
2. Important Points for Viva/MCQs   4–39
3. General Pharmacology   40–53
4. CVS   54–77
5. Endocrinology   78–82
6. Chemotherapy   83–138
7. Newer Questions   139–146

FACTUAL DATA

* Sumitriptan and ergotamine should not be administered within **24** hours of each other :

* **Half life of Aensine in blood is** 10 sec.

* **After stopping disulfiram, sensitization to alcohol lasts for** 7-14 days

* **Fentanyl-droperidol are usually used in fixed combination of** 0.05, 2.5 **mg respectively :**

* **Pregnancy should be avoided even after withdrawal of gold therapy upto** 6 months

* Half life of Urokinase is **15-20** min :

* Surgery is contraindicated in a patient on thrombolytic therapy for **10 days**

* t-PA (Tissue Plasminogen activator) is a serine protease containing 527 amino acid residues with half life of about **5-10 min**

* Plasma half life of Ondansetron is **3-4** hours :

* Rifabutin acts on **RNA polymerase**

* Dose of selegiline higher than **10** mg may induce inhibition of MAO-A :

* **After stopping Omeprazole, acid secretion begins within** 3-5 days

* **Half life of Atleplase is** 3-4 min

* Half life of adenosine is **10 sec.**

* Rifabulin, an antitubercular drug, has a mean terminal half life of **45** hours.

* Moricizine is a new, class **1** antiarrythmic drug :

* ↓ **QT interval** is a cardiac effect of Lidocaine
* Peak effect of Quabain is in **1—2 hours**
* Dose of glycopyrrolate is -mgI/M as preanesthetic **0.1-0.3**
* **When given to a patient on phenytoin, dose of theophylline should be** 1.5 **times :**
* Famotidine is excreted unchanged in urine as **70** % .
* Roxatidine is **2** times as potent as ranitidine.
* Famolidine is **20** times more potent than cimeticdine and **8** times more potent that ranitidine respectively.
* Effect of Esmolol lasts for **15-20 min** min.
* **12-15 hours** is true about plasma half life of Tocainide.
* Duration of action of Warfarin is **4-7 days.**
* Duration of action of astemizole is about hours Dimenhydrinate **72.**
* Elimination halfife of clavulanic acid is **1 hour**
* 1 C.C. of buprenorphine injection contains **—0.3** mg.
* Cardiac glycosides increase automaticity i.e. phase **4.**
* Ondansetron mainly antagonises **5 HT.**
* Time of onset of prompt insulin zinc suspension is **60 min**
* The incidence of nasal allergy in aspirin users is 1-2%.
* Penicillin was first used for systemic infections in 1941.
* The half life of intravenous plain insulin is 5-7 min.
* In cotrimoxazole, sulphamethoxazole and triomethoprin are in ratio of 5 : 1.
* Dexamethasone is **30 times** potent than cortisone.
* Half life phenytoin - 24 to 36 hours.
* Digitalis should be stopped 48 hours before electroversion.
* Therapeutic serum level of digoxin—0.8 to 1.6 ng/ml.
* Half life of Adenosone in blood is 10 sec.
* After stopping Omeprazole, acid secretion begins within 3-5 days.

* Half life of Atleplase is 3-4 min.

* The dose of a drug for an infant less than 2 years old is obtained by multiplying the child's age in months by the adult dose and dividing the result by 150 is **Fried's rule.**

* Half life of Urokinase is **15-20 min.**

* Time of onset of prompt insulin zinc suspension is 60 min.

* Surgery is contraindicated for **10 days** in a patient on thrombolytic therapy.

* t-PA (Tissue Plasmonogen activator) is a serine protease containing **527** amino acid residues with half life of about **5-10 min.**

* Deafness, epigastric pain and insomnia are sideeffects of Tolmetin.

* Plasma half life of Ondansetron is **3-4 hours.**

* **Rifabulin**, an antitubercular drug, has a mean terminal half life of **45 hours.**

IMPORTANT POINTS FOR VIVA/MCQ'S

* Riboflavin deficiency predisposes to snow blindness.

* Botulinum toxin produces respiratory paralysis, tetanus toxin produces muscular spasm and convulsions, diphtheria toxin damages the heart and the toxins of staphylococci rupture RBC's

* Tolbutamide metabolism is **inhibited** by phenylbutazone, coumarin anticoagulants, chloramphenicol and sulfonamides, hence hypoglycaemia may ensure.

* Phenytoin metabolism is **inhibited** by coumarin anticoagulants, INH (slow acetylers), phenylbutazone, cimetidine, disulfiram & sulthiame so that phenytoin intoxication may occur.

* **Vancomycin** is the drug of first choice (DOIC) against clostridium difficile

* Amantadine is the DOIC used against Influenza 'A' whereas Ribavirin is the DOIC used against the Respiratory syncytial virus.

* Thiopentone, Phenoxybeazamine and Organophosphate poisons are highly fat soluble, hence stored in fat.

* Sulfomethoxine, phenylbutazone, warfar and clofibrate are highly bound to protein.

* Higher the therapeutic index, safer is the drug. eg Penicillin has got high therapeutic index. Digitalis has got low therapeutic index.

* Paul Ehrlich is regarded as the **father of modern chemotherapy.**

* Penicillin was discovered by **Alexander Fleming** whereas the therapeutic use of Penicillin was demonstrated by **Florrey and Chain.**

* L-dopa is not effective against drug induced Parkinsonism, in such cases anticholinergic drugs are effective.

* Chlorpromazine produces hypothermia, so useful in hyperpyrexia.

* Oxyethazine (a local anaesthetic) is used with gastric antacids to reduce the peptic ulcer pain.

* The most potent available nonsteroid anti inflammatory drug is indomethacin.

* Sulindac is a prodrug, so are lisinopril and enalapril.

* Probenecid is a uricosuric drug.

* The nicotinic I receptor is present in a autonomic ganglia whereas nicotinic II in skeletal muscles.

* The antidote for beta-bloclers is isoprenaline (10mg) sublingually or by inhalation.

* Guanethidine is the most potent of the adrenergic neurone blocking drugs.

* Morphine increases ADH and reduces urinary output.

* Heparin is commercially from Ox lung.

* H1 (Histamine receptors are located in bronchi and intestines while H2 (Histamine) receptors in the stomach whereas both are located in the blood vessels.

* Thiazolylamine is H1 receptor agonists whereas Betazol and Dimaprit are H2 receptor agonists.

* Levamisole is a drug that acts on macrophages and enhances phagocytosis.

* Penicillins and Cephlosporins together are called beta lactum antibiotics.

* Mecillinam is a newer penicillin useful against salmonella and shigella.

* Thiaenamycin is a beta lactam antibiotic that inhibits both bacterial cell wall synthesis and beta lactamase.

* Fusidic acid is a steroid antibiotic.

* INH and Rifampicins are the most potent antikoch's drug.

* Red blood cells acts as depo for ethambutol

* Streptozotocin is used in insulinoma.

* Methandienone is predominantly anabolic and least androgenic.

* Reports indicate the invitro anti-HIV activity of HPA-23, inferferon alpha, foscamet and zidovudine.

* Zidovudine (AZT) and Didanosine are licensed drugs in AIDS patients.

* Morphine is **contraindicated** in bronchial asthma.

* Ethambutol is **contraindicated** in children and may cause visual field defects (blue vision).

* Treatment of choice in trigeminal neuralgia is carbamazepine.

* **Best** route to give steroids in steroid dependent asthmatic is inhalation.

* **Drug of choice** in a case of acute MI with arrythmias is lignocaine.

* **Hypersensitive cholestatic jaundice** is due to erythromycin estolate.

* Beta blockers are **contraindicated** in bronchial asthma and CHF.

* **Lactational failure** may occur with bromocriptine.

* **Drug of choice** in hypertension with dissection of aorta is sodium nitroprusside.

* ACE inhibitors (Enalapril, Lisinopril) may cause cough.

* **Drug of choice** in gonococcal and angioneurotic oedema infection is penicillin.

* Leukoencephalopathy is seen with use of vincristine.

* Effect of dopamine on kidney may be blocked by propranolol.

* Plasma expanders with oxygen carrying capacity are **fluorocarbons.**

* Lisinopril is **contraindicated** in bilateral renal artery stenosis.

* **Hypogeusia** is seen with use of captopril.

* Calcium channel blockers with predominant peripheral effects in nifedipine.

* **Haemorrhagic** cystitis is caused by cyclophosphamide.

* PAPP is used in treatment of poisoning with cyanide.

* Photosensitivity is caused by phenothiazines e.g. chlorpromazine.

* **Pseudomembranous** colitis is associated with clindamycin.

* Most serious side effect of streptomycin is impairment of vestibular function.

* **Dimercaprol** is indicated in treatment of poisoning due to mercury.
* **Commonest** side effect of oral iron therapy is GI disturbances.
* A drug which is a direct inhibitor of bacterial nucleic acid synthesis is rifampicin.
* Efficacy of oral contraceptives is decreased with concurrent use of rifampicin.
* **Metaphase arrest** is caused by vincristine.
* **Jarisch-Hexhemer reaction** is associated with penicillin and syphilis.
* Macrolide **contraindicated** in lactation is spiramycin.
* **Drug of choice** in hepatolenticular degeneration is penicillamine.
* Lithium is **contraindicated** in kidney failure.
* Drug best used in toxoplasmosis is **spiramycin.**
* Morphine causes vomiting by acting on CIZ.
* Theophylline levels in blood are **increased** by erythromycin.
* Resistance to antitubercular drugs develop by **mutation.**
* **Pentamidine** is used in AIDS.
* Enalapril is a **prodrug.**
* Beta blocker without LA effect is **timolol.**
* Propranolol is **contraindicated** in Diabetes mellitus.
* **Drug of choice** is acute anaphylaxis is adrenaline.
* Aspirin is **contraindicated** in a patient on warfarin.
* G-6-P-D deficiency protects against falciparum malaria.
* Guenethidine is **contraindicated** in pheochromocytoma whereas labeltolol may be used.
* Propylthiouracil inhibits coupling of iodotyrosines.
* Drug used in **dissolving gall bladder stone** is chenodeoxycholic acid.
* Drug causing folate deficiency are cotrimoxazole and methotrexate.
* Phenytoin causes deficiency of vitamin C,D and folate.

* Side effect of Diloxanide furonate is flatulance.
* **Drug of choice** in status epilepticus is Diazepam.
* **Hyperplasia of gums** is a side effect of phenytoin.
* INH is metabolized by acetylation and may cause peripheral neuritis (Pyridoxine deficiency) and liver toxicity.
* **Pulmonary fibrosis** may be caused by bleomycin, nitrofurantoin and amiodarone.
* **Pseudolymphoma** is a side effect of treatment with phenytoin.
* **Drug of choice** in diabetes insipidus is desmopressin.
* Thymosin is an **immunostimulant** drug.
* Glomerular damage may be caused by penicillamine toxicity.
* **Optic neuritis** may be caused by chloroquine.
* **treatment of choice** in methanol induced optic neuritis is NaHCO3.
* In **acute MI,** the drug of choice is streptokinase.
* Aplastic anaemia is a side effect of chloramphenicol.
* **Budesonide** is a new bronchodilator.
* **Hyperprolactinemia** is a side effect of metoclopramide and neuroleptics.
* 6 mercaptopurine potentiates the action of allopurinol.
* **Treatment of choice** in Wegner's granulomatosis is cyclophosphamide.
* Antidepressant producing extrapyramidal side effect is amoxapine.
* Lithium is absolutely contraindicated in pregnancy and lactation.
* Teratogenic effect of lithium is **Ebstein's anomaly.**
* **Drug of choice** in cryptococal meningitis is amphotericin B.
* Drug of choice in **Prinzmetal angina** is Diltiazem.
* Quinidine is **contraindicated** in digoxin toxicity.
* Drug which reduces afterload but not preload is hydralazine.
* **Antidote** of amantia muscaria is atropine.
* Sodium cromoglycate stabilized mast cells.

* Adriamycin is a cardiotoxic drug.
* Hypersensitivity hepatitis is caused by nicotinic acid.
* Primaquin is not used as primary tissue schizonticidal.
* Oestrogen acts through intracytoplasmic receptors.
* **Drug of choice** in acute gout is colchicine.
* Pentoxifyline is **contraindicated** in acute MI, pregnancy and massive retinal haemorrhages.
* **Ofloxacin** is a new fluorinated quinolone.
* Alopecia may be caused by sodium valproate, fluoxetine and lithium.
* **Drug useful** in alopecia is Minoxidil.
* Virilization in Stein Levinthal syndrome is due to increased secretion of ovarian androgens.
* **Pseudomembrane colitis** may be caused by ceftriaxone.
* The molecule which releases TSH from pituitary is glycopeptide.
* **Dapsone** is used in leprosy, madura foot and dermatitis herpetiformis.
* **Zero order kinetics** is seen with phenytoin, ethanol and salicytates.
* Diphenindione is the **longest** acting antihistaminic.
* Flu like syndrome may be a side effect of rifampicin.
* **Least hepatotoxic antitubercular** drug is ethambutol and streptomycin does not have hepatotoxicity.
* **Selegilline** is useful in Parkinsonism and Depression.
* Lugol's iodine inhibits the iodine uptake.
* Drug **most useful** in digitalis induced arrythmia is phenytoin.
* Digoxin is eliminated from body by glomerular filtration.
* **Drug of choice** in ulcerative colitis is salazopyrin.
* **Cyclosporia-A** is useful in aplastic anaemia.
* **Painful Gynaecomastia** is caused by cimetidine.
* Drug with extensive first bypass metabolism is propranolol.
* Antacids decrease the absorption of tetracycline, ofloxacin, ketoconazole and iron.

* **Drug of choice** in chronic recalcitrant cystic acne is retinoids.
* Tetracycline may be given in renal failure is doxycycline.
* Demeclocycline may cause **photosensitivity.**
* Fusidic acid is a steroidal antibiotic.
* Acetazolamide is used in Petitmal epilepsy, glaucoma, peptic ulcer and as a diuretic.
* For quick and vigorous diuresis, **diuretic of choice** is frusemide.
* Neomycin use may cause malabsorption syndrome on prolonged use.
* **Flupenthixol** is an antipsychotic drug with antidepressant property.
* Pyruvium pamoate is used in the treatment of enterobiasis.
* **Drug of choice** in Addison's disease is hydrocortisone.
* Short duration of action of thiopentone is due to **redistribution.**
* Probenecid **increases** the levels of penicillin.
* Tannic acid is a good example of astringent.
* **Drug of choice** in Diphtheria is penicillin.
* **Drug of choice** in multiple myeloma is melphalan.
* Most useful drug in the management of hypertension due to pheochromocytoma is phenoxybenzamine.
* Most powerful emetic agent is morphine.
* TCE (Tetrachloroethylene) is used in the treatment of ankylostomiasis.
* **Master's test** is employed to evaluate antianginal drugs.
* **Most serious** side efect of phenylbutazone is agranulocytosis.
* **Drug of choice** in cardiogenic shock is I/V dopamine.
* Drug useful in **anovulatory infertility** is clomiphene.
* **Drug of choice** in Paget's disease is calcitonin.
* A patient with anosmia will respond to inhalation of liquor ammonia.
* Alcohol is metabolized by oxidation.
* **Safest** anaesthetic agent is N2O.

* Most important toxicity of phenacetin is renal damage.
* Intraluminal **amoebicide** of choice is diloxanide.
* Danthron acts as a purgative due to irritant action.
* Drug of choice in ventricular tachycardia is lignocaine.
* Colistin is closely related to polymyxin.
* **Drug of choice** in CML is Busulphan.
* **Myopathy** is caused by alcohol, lithium, salbutamol and steroids.
* Labetolol is both alpha and beta blocker.
* Penicillin acts on cell wall.
* Barbiturates are **contraindicated** in prophyria.
* **Antidote** of tubocurare is neostigmine.
* **Drug of choice** in non-rheumatoid arthritis is indomethacin.
* **Drug of choice** in Juvenile rheumatoid arthritis is aspirin.
* **Drug of choice** in acute migraine is ergotamine or a new drug sumitriptan whereas in prophylaxis flunarizine, propranolol, amitriptyline, cyprohepatadine or calcium channel blockers are useful.
* **SLE like rash** may be seen with hydralazine, procainamide and INH.
* **Omeprazole** causes negative gastric acid pump.
* Digoxin is not used in CHF caused due to aortic stenosis.
* Most readily absorbed oral cardiac glycoside is digitoxin.
* Urinary excretion of probenecid can be enhanced by administration of sodium bicarbonate .
* Metal useful in rheumatoid arthritis is gold.
* Dose of 6-mercapatopurine requires reduction with allopurinol.
* **Drug of choice** in treatment of herpes simplex keratitis is topical acyclovir.
* **Drug of choice** in drug induced parkinsonism is anticholinergic antihistaminic.
* **Didanosine** may caused pancreatitis.
* **Drug of choice** in petitmal epilepsy is ethosuximide.

* **Dales vasomotor reversal phenomenon** is seen with adrenaline.
* Disulfiram like reaction may be seen with metronidazole, "griseozulvin.
* Thioridazine may cause pigmentary retinopathy.
* Amikacin is ototoxic.
* Noscapine is antitussive.
* Pyrazinamide increases uric acid levels.
* Ergotamine is used in acute migraine because it causes vasoconstriction.
* **INH toxicity** is treated by Gastric lavage and Pyridoxine I/V (dose by dose).
* Diethylcarbazine is used in filariasis.
* Treatment of choices of non-specific urethritis is tetra cycline.
* Streptokinase is used in acute MI.
* Hemolytic anaemia may be a side effect of methyldopa.
* Penicillamine, tridione and gold may lead to nephrotic syndrome.
* Ingestion of liver of polar bear may caue of acute poisoning of vitamin A.
* Aspirin toxicity may cause respiratory alkalosis and metabolic acidosis.
* Strychnine acts on postsynaptic block.
* **Drug of choice** in breast cancer is cyclophosphamide.
* **Tachyphylaxis** is seen with ephedrine.
* Triiodothyronine is **most rapidly acting** thyroid preparation.
* **Antidote** of heparin is protamine sulphate.
* **Antidote** of warfarin is fresh saline and Vitamin K1.
* **Treatment of choice** in thalassemia is desferroxamine.
* Nifedipine is used in hypertension, angina and Gilles de la Tourette syndrome.
* Timolol reduces intraocular pressure by a reduction in aqueous humor production
* Most effective drug in seronegative ankylosing spondylosis in aspirin.

* Vitamin resembling a hormone is Vitamin D.
* Therapeutic use of acetylcholine is not possible because it is rapidly degraded.
* **Treatment of choice** of Hypsarrythmia is ACTH.
* Nalidixic acid is used in UTI.
* Term '**soporofic**' is synonymous with hypnotic.
* Treatment of choice in Burkitt's lymphoma is cyclophosphamide.
* Osteoporosis may be caused by corticosteroids.
* Pilocarpine is **best used** in chronic simple glaucoma.
* Diazoxide is a vasodilator.
* Sodium cromoglycate acts by decreasing autocoid secretion.
* Steroids are used to stop fibrosis.
* **Drug of choice** in myoclonus is clonezepam.
* MAO inhibitors are **contraindicated** with tricyclic antidepressants.
* MAO inhibitors should not be given with pethidine.
* Morphine like rash is seen with INH.
* Drug useful in **Dracunculosis** is Niridazole.
* Pancreatitis may be caused by alcohol, steroids and diuretics.
* **Bromocriptine** is used in Parkinsonism, acromegaly and infertility.
* **Nimodipine** is a calcium channel blocker decreases vascular spasm in Ischaemic stroke.
* Penicillin was given by Flemming. streptomycin by Waksman and Erythromycin by McGurie.
* Phenytoin may produce nystagmus, ataxia and osteomalacia.
* Ether produces **greatest** degree of muscular relaxation.
* Dose of digoxin is reduced in old age, hepatic impairment and hypokalemia.
* **Danazol** is useful in amenorrhoea endometricosis and fibroadenosis
* Medical adrenalectomy is produced by aminoglulethimide.

* Paracetamol is N-acetyl-p-aminophenol.

* Captopril inhibits conversion of angiotensin I to II.

* Drug used to treat Alzheimer's disease is tetrahydro-aminacrine.

* Atropine poisoning is **best** antagonised by physostigmine.

* Chlorpromazine causes obstructive Jaundice.

* **Bleomycin** primarily affects lungs (pulm. fibrosis).

* Hypoglycemia is least likely with tolbutamide.

* Reserpine produces **suicidal depression.**

* Aminophylline may cause convulsions.

* Physostigmine crosses blood brain barrier whereas neostigmine does not.

* Cisplatin is effective in treatment of testicular carcinoma.

* Rifampicin inhibits bacterial nucleic acid synthesis.

* The **cumulative dose limiting toxicity** of adriamycin is cardiomyopathy.

* Host response to antimicrobial therapy is influenced by hepatic and renal function, age and genetic background.

* **Clozapine.** a newer antipsychotic, has the fatal side effect of agranulocytosis.

* **Ritodrine hydrochloride** is used in the treatment of premature labour.

* **Drug of choice** in curare poisoning is neostigmine.

* Dihydrostreptomycin is toxic to auditory branch of 8th nerve.

* Propranolol is useful in Thyrotoxicosis, Hypertension, Arrythmias, Pheochromocytoma, Angina and Digitalis toxicity (Mnemonic **'THAPAD'.**

* **Clavulanic acid** is an irreversible inhibitor of beta lactamase.

* Phenytoin may cause cerebellar syndrome.

* Cisplatin is not a cell cycle specific antineoplastic drug.

* Ibuprofen mainly inhibits the prostaglandin synthetase.

* The **earliest toxic symptom** of digitalis toxicity is anorexia, nausea, vomiting.

* Iodohydroxy quinoline causes submyelo optic neuropathy (SMON).

* **Drug useful** in vaccinia is methisazone.

* Forced diuresis is **most useful** in poisoning due to phenobarbitone.

* Melphalan is a **radiomimetic** drug.

* Metronidazole is used in Gram negative septicemia, giardiasis, amoebiasis and trichomoniasis.

* Aluminium hydroxide causes constipation whereas magnesium salts cause diarrhoea.

* Drug with **antiandrogenic effects** is cyproterone acetate.

* Amphetamines are used in hyperkinetic syndrome and narcolepsy.

* Amantadine acts by increasing dopamine levels.

* **Fenfluramine** is used in obesity.

* Rifampicin increases metabolism of oral contraceptives.

* **Antidote** of aniline dye is methylene blue.

* **Drug of choice** in actinomycosis is penicillin.

* Cimetidine is **most useful** in duodenal ulcer.

* **Antidote** of oral silver nitrate poisoning is normal saline.

* Morphine is **contraindicated** in head injury.

* Sudden stoppage of clonidine may cause rebound hypertension.

* Clonidine is useful in hypertension and opiate withdrawal.

* Reserpine may cause suicidal depression.

* **tardive dyskinesia** may result due to longterm use of neuroleptics and an antidepressant, amoxapine.

* **Clozapine,** a newer neuroleptic, does not cause tardive dyskinesia, extrapyramidal syndrome and neuroleptic syndrome.

* Tricyclic antidepressants are **contraindicated** in glaucoma.

* Treatment of choice in Parkinsonism is L-dopa.

* **Drug of choice** in Paroxysmal Atrial tachycardia is calcium channel blocker.

* Papaverine injection (locally) is used in **erectile impotence** (organic type).

* **Naltrexone** is used in opiate dependence.

* **Flumazenil** is benzodiazepine antagonist (reverses sedation).

* **Moclobemide** is a MAO-B inhibitor antidepressant.

* Thioridazine causes minimum extrapyramidal effects among phenothiazines.

* **Amineptin** is an antidepressant.

* Non-sedating antidepressants are fluoxetine, paroxetine, Amineptin and Nortriptyline.

* Digitalis was discovered by **William Withering.**

* **Drug of choice** for brucellosis is Tetracycline.

* **Drug useful** in Postoperative urinary retention is Bethanecol.

* **Drug of choice** in acute angina is nitroglycerine.

* Triamterene and spironolactone act on distal tubule.

* Oral hypoglycemic with **longest duration** of action is chlorpropamide.

* Phenothiazines may precipitate diabetes mellitus.

* Drugs useful in **nocturnal enuresis** are tricyclic antidepressants (Imipramine) and desmopressin.

* Antibacterial spectrum of penicillin most closely resembles that of bacitracin.

* Pyridoxine is **contraindicated** with L-dopa therapy.

* Insulin can be given I/V is crystalline zinc insulin.

* The world's oldest pharmacology or therapeutic writings evolve from India and China.

* The earliest Indian records on Indian pharmacopia are from the Vedas (Rigveda 3000 BC).

* "PAN TASO" (Chinese materia medica) contained many herbal, vegetable and metallic, as well as few animal products having pharmacological actions (2735 BC).

* The earliest sources of Western Medicine come from Egypt and Assyria & Babylonia.

* The **Papyrus** discovered by Eber in 1872 was made in 1500 BC, mentioned about 700 herbal products including opium.

* **Paul Ehrlich** (1854-1915) known as father of modern chemotherapy.

  * demonstrated (1891) the efficacy of methylene blue in the T/t of human malaria.

  * synthesized various arsenical compounds effective against syphilis and other spirochaetal infections.

  * introduced the term chemotherapeutic index (a ratio of the maximum tolerated dose of a drug to its minimum curative dose).

  Note : Now-a-days chemotherapeutic index has been replaced by therapeutic index LD50/ED50.

  * introduced arsephrenamine-Ist really effective chemotherapeutic agent in man, in the I/t of syphilis.

  * was awarded Noble Prize in (1909).

* **Domagk, Mietsch &** their colleagues (1938) demonstrated the efficacy of Prontosil (a dye with a sulfonamide side chain).

* Prontosil inhibits growth of streptococci both in vitro & vivo.

* Methyldopa causes reversible hemolytic anaemia.

* Side effects of cyclosporins—Nephrotoxicity.

* Original and most active Penicillin—Benzyl penicillin.

* Probenecid will raise the blood level of penicillin by delaying its excretion by kidney.

* Clavulinic acid—a new beta-lactem agent. It is a potent inhibitor of many beta lactamases.

* The commonest adverse effect of Tetracycline—Diarrhoea.

* The tetracycline that can be given in Renal failure—Doxycycline.

* The commonest adverse effect of the aminoglycoides is in the eighth cranial nerve.

* The commonest adverse effect of the aminoglycoides is in the eighth cranial nerve.

* i) Kanamycin tends ot cause deafness first. ii) With Gentamycin and streptomycin—the vestibular division affected first -causes vertigo.

* The ototoxicity of the aminoglycosides is related to the age of the patient, the serum level, and the duration of administration.

* Chloramphenicol causes — Bone marrow Aplasia.
* Principal side effects of erythromycin—Diarrhoea.
* The most common indication for the use of sulphonamides is cystitis.
* Sulphonamides can detach protein bound drugs such as warfarin and sulphonyl urea antidiabetic agents and there by cause overdosage.
* Sulphonamides should not be used topically.
* High dose cotrimoxazole is used to treat pneumonia caused by pneumocystis carinii
* Metronidazole should not be given to women during the first trimester of pregnancy.
* Alcohol should be avoided during therapy with metronidazole.
* Flucytosine is active only against yeasts.
* Griseofulvin is selectively concentrated in keratin.
* Drug of choice for widespread or chronic dematophyte infections—Griseofulvin.
* The only notable adverse reaction of Acyclovir being a rise in serum urea if the intravenous injection is given too quickly.
* Amiloride and trimeterene are not aldosterone antagonists.
* Triameterene when given with indomethacin it may cause acute renal failure.
* Drug for treatment of addisonian crisis—Hydrocortisone.
* Mannitol delays acute Renal failure in Septicaemia shock.
* Fibrinolytic drug—Streptokinase.
* **Drugs which inhibit platelet aggregation**
    * Dipyridamole
    * Hydroxychloroquine
    * Aspirin
* **Appetite suppressants**
    * Amphetamine
    * Dextroamphetamine
    * Fenfluramine

* Mithramycin—lower the calcium levels.

* Methysergide is serotonin antagonist.

* **Contraindications to ergotamine**
  * Septic or infectious states
  * Peripheral vascular disease
  * Coronary disease
  * Pregnancy
  * Thyrotoxicosis

* Action of Tricyclic antidepressants—Facilitation of Mononinoneuro-transmit tears by inhibition of transmitter reuptake.

* Side effects of propranolol—lethargy, insomnia, constipation.

* Betahistine, a vasodilator has been used successfully in some cases of Meniere's disease.

* Patients suffering from cholera or cholera like gastroenteritis should be treated with tetracycline while infection due to compylobacter responds to erythromycin.

* The astringents, because of their ability to precipitate superficial proteins, form a protective layer on the mucous membrane.

* Lactobacillus acidophilus used in treatment of certain chronic diarrhoeas.

* Bisacodyl is laxative.

* Histamine is used to test the maximum ability of the stomach to secrete hydrochloric acid (Kay's augmented histamine stimulation test).

* Aluminium hydroxide-constipation is the major adverse effect.

* Milk of Magnesia contains Magnesium hydroxide.

* Omeprazole inhibit gastric acid (Proton) pump.

* Omeprazole is also effective in Zollinger Ellison syndrome.

* Ergot alkaloids increase the tone of the cervix in contrast to oxytocin which decreases it.

* Ethacridine lactate used extra-amniotically for second trimester abortion.

* Sulfonamides enhance the anticoagulant potency of warfarin.
* Penicillins mainly absorbed from the duodenum.
* Erythromycin is the drug of choice in diarrhoea due to compylobacter jejuni and preumonia due to Legionella.
* Streptomycin exhibit synergism with Penicillin.
* Streptomycin-Penicillin combination useful in treatment of bacteremia and endocarditis duct to strep. faecalis.
* Drug useful in treatment of Tularemia - Streptomycin.
* Paraomycin (Aminoglycoside) also shows considerable activity against E. histolytica.
* Cefozidime and Cefsulodin are the only cephalosphorins highly active against pseud. aeruginosa.
* Chloramphenicol can be relatively safely administered in patients with renal impairment.
* Griseofulvin is not effective against candida.
* Only rifampicin acts against persisters of tuberculous bacilli.
* Streptomycin is bactericidal against tubercle bacilli rapidly multiplying at Neutral pH in the walls of tuberculous cavities, but does not penetrate into the macrophages nor into caseous material.
* **Pyrazinamide**
    * It is effective only against tubercle bacilli within macrophage.
    * Achieves a concentration in CSF almost equal to Plasma levels.
* One of the side effects of cycloserine-convulsions.
* Chloroquine—is used only in extra intestinal amoebiasis.
* The commones side effect of Diloxanide furoate is — Flatulence.
* Radioactive gold is used as a palliate measure in the treatment of malignant pleural and peritoneal effusions.
* Drug of choice for acute lymphatic leukemia—Vincristine with prednisolone.
* Teratogenic effect of Thalidomide—limb abnormalities (Seal limbs).
* Atropine causes cycloplegia and mydriasis persists for a week.

* Heparin is a strongly acidic compound.
* The urinary ketone test may be falsely positive in patients in valproic acid.
* Infantile spasm are best treated with ACTH.
* Codeine is often used as substitute during treatment of Methadone addiction.
* Doxapram is a respiratory stimulant.
* The most common adverse effect of indomethacin is headache.
* **Drugs causing cataracts :**
  * Phenothiazines
  * Corticosteroids
  * Busulfan
  * Chlorambucil
* Cimetidine and INH inhibit the hepatic microsomal enzymes.
* In severe cases of depression with delusions, suicidal ideations and remissions—ECT is preferred to drug therapy (Electro convulsive therapy).
* The drug omeprazole-inhibit Gastric H+ - K+ ATPase (Proton Pump)
* Sucralfate forms adherent protein complexes at the peptic ulcer site.
* Proglumide blocks the Gastric receptors.
* Pirenzepine (Anti cholinergic drug)-block the M1, muscarinic, receptors.
* Cimetidine, Ranitidine-Block the H2 receptors.
* Nicotinic acid is useful in all forms of hyperlipoproteinemias except type I.
* Copper deficiency causes anemia.
* The symptom that responds first to Levodopa in Parkinsonism— Akinesia.
* Aminoglycosides may exacerbate Myasthenia gravis.
* Aminoglycoside antibiotics may produce a clinical disturbance similar to botulism by preventing the release of acetylcholine from nerve endings.

* Commonest side effects of Carbamazepine — Drowsiness.
* **Teratogenic effects of Anti convulsant drugs**
  * Cleft lip, spina bifida, cardiac defects etc.
  * Risk is greatest during the first trimester
  * Carbamazepine may be less teratogenic than other agents.
* The most important clinical indicator of phenytoin toxicity — Ataxia.
* Levels of phenobarbital may rise after initiation of valproic acid therapy.
* Therapeutic levels of which antiepileptic drug are poorly defined for Sodium valproate.
* **Cytotoxic drug causing Alopecia**
  * Adriamycin
  * Cyclophosphamide
* Adriamycin is associated with risk of developing cardiac failure.
* Cisplatin causes a progressive impairment of renal function.
* Aminoglutethamide inhibits the enzyme—Desmolase.
* Treatment of choice of ventricular tachycardia in urgent cases is intravenous lignocaine.
* Cardioversion should be avoided if digitalis toxicity is the cause of ventricular tachycardia.
* **Drugs that can be used for both atrial and ventricular arrythmias**
  * Procainamide
  * Quinidine
  * Disopyramide
* Disopyramide has weak atropine like effects and may cause urinary retention or precipitate glaucoma.
* Cardioselective Beta blockers—Metoprolol, Atenolol.
* **One of the side effects of**
  * Amiodarone—Corneal deposits
  * Quinidine—Diarrhoea
  * Verapamil—Constipation
  * Mediletine—Ataxia

* In circulatory failure, the most effective antidote to renal vasoconstriction is low dose dopamine.
* Digoxin toxicity is potentiated by hypokalemia.
* The drug causing pulmonary arterial hypertension — fenfluramine.
* Drug for intracoronary thrombolysis—Streptokinase, urikinase.
* Side effect of Guanethidine—Postural hypertension
* Drugs-Quinidine, procainamide, Tricyclics cause Prolonged QT interval.
* Digitalis toxicity may be precipitated by hypokalemia hypoxemia, hypercalcemia.
* Digitalis is contraindicated in Acute myocardial infarction, Acute myocarditis, heart blood ventricular tachycardia.
* Hypertension is not a contraindication to the use of Digitalis.
* Earliest ECG changes of Digitalis toxicity—Depression scooping out of ST segment.
* Digitalis therapy should be stopped immediately if toxicity is suspected.
* **Side effects of verapamil**
  * Decreased left ventricular function
  * Constipation
  * Increased serum digoxin level
* Atrial natriuretic peptide has potent vasodilatory and natriuretic properties.
* In some patients ACE-inhibitors cause cough possible via an immunological reaction.
* Vasodilator therapy (e.g Captopril) is not indicated in congestive heart failure due to Aortic stenosis. Because they cause a serious fall in Blood pressure.
* Nitroglycerin may precipitate chest pain in — Hypertrophic obstructive cardiomyopathy.
* Dialysis dementia is caused by —Aluminium toxicity.
* Cotrimoxazole is not useful for syphilis.

* Chloroquine do not cause photosensitivity.
* d-tubocurarine does not cross the placenta or Blood brain barrier.
* Digoxin toxicity when the serum levels are more than —2.4 ng/ml.
* The therapeutic serum level of Lithium—0.6 to 1.2 mmol/l.
* Slow inactivation of Isoniazid is due to Molecular abnormality of —Isoniazid acetylase in Liver.
* Suxamethonium sensitivity is due to molecular abnormality of —Pseudochlinesterase in Plasma.
* Chlorpropamide enhance the action of ADH on distal nephron.
* Drugs useful in Rx of SIADH—Demeclocycline (a tetracycline derivative)
* Demeclocycline inhibits the action of ADH on the collecting duct.
* **Drugs causing Nephrogenic diabetes insipidus**
    * Lithium
    * Demeclocycline
* One of the complications due to insulin—Presbyopia.
* Chlorpropamide causes facial flushing after ingestion of alcohol.
* Chromium deficiency causes insulin resistance.
* **Drugs also useful in treatment of Diabetes insipidus**
    * Clofibrate—increase vasopressin secretion
    * Chlorpropamide—increases the renal response to vasopressin
* Glucogon exerts its effect on glucose output via a protein kinase that inhibits glycogen synthesis, facilities glycogenolysis, and inhibits conversion of phosphoenol pyruvate to pyruvate.
* Drugs that inhibit insulin secretion—Diazoxide, Thiazide, diuretics.
* Biguanides do not affect insulin secretion but increase glucose utilisation. They increase anaerobic glycolysis within the cells. They also decrease glucose absorption from the gastrointestinal tract.
* Metyrapone inhibits Adrenal 11β-Hydroxylase.

* The effective dose of amphotericin and thus its toxic effects of the kidney, can be reduced by combining it with flucytosine.

* Nasal spray available for **Allergic Rhinitis** are
  * Sodium chromoglycate nasal spray
  * Beclomethasone dipropionate nasal spray
  * Budenoside nasal spray

* Drug for treatment of **Hamman Rich syndrome** — Corticosteroids.

* Side effect of Nasal insuffiation of pituitary snuff in Diabetes insipidus — Allergic Alveolitis.

* Bile salts increase the flow as well as concentration of bile and hence, are termed choleretics.

* Chenodeoxycholic acid dissolves **radiolucent gallstones**.

* Nitrous oxide was discovered by **Priestly**.

* Steroid anaesthetic is **Althesin**.

* Diethyl ether is extremely soluble in blood.

* Halothane causes hypotension.

* Ether does not sensitize the myocardium to adrenaline.

* Cautery cannot be used along with ether anaesthesia.

* Halothane employed to induce controlled hypotension to provide a "**Bloodless field**".

* Halothane anaesthetic is preferred in patients with history of bronchial asthma.

* Nitrous oxide is probably the **safest** of the anaesthetic agents.

* Aluminium poisoning in patients with renal failure who are receiving dialysis treatment causes a rapidly progressive dementia that resembles Alzheimer's disease.

* Use of benzyl benzoate is **contraindicated** on broken and abraded skin and also in presence of secondary infections

* Use of silver sulfadiazine is **contraindicated** in pregnant women, premature infants and infants below 2 years

* With enalapril, there is steep fall in blood pressure on first dose

* Amiodarone is **contraindicated** in sinus bradycarnia, SA or AV block, iodine sensitivity, thyroid dysfunction, pregnancy and lactation

* Streptokinase is **contraindicated** in aortic dissection

* Ferrous sulphate decreases absorption of levodopa, penicillamine and ciprofloxacin

* Folic acid is **contraindicated** in imprecisely diagnosed megaloblastic anemia and malignancy

* Enalapril causes neutropenia and altered taste sensation

* Bromocriptine is useful in acromegaly

* Selegiline is **contraindicated** in convulsive disorders and in children. Special precaution is to be taken in psychosis, cardiac arrythmias and angina.

* Penicillamine is **contraindicated** in patients on gold therapy and anlimalarials

* Amiodarone increases effects of diagoxin, warfarin, beta blockess, quinidine, procainamide, encainide, flecainide, diltiazem

* Aluminium hydroxide, ethanol, phenytoin, phenobarb, rifampicin decreases effect of atenolol. NSAIDs oppose antihypertensive effect of atenolol whereas digitalis and verapamil enhances cardiac depressant effect. Hypoglycermide effect of sulfonylureas is attenuated by atenolol whereas response to adrenaline in anaphylaxis is reduced.

* Cefotaxime, ceftazidime and cephalexin are contraindicated in porphyria

* Plasma concentrations of glibenclamide are increased with ACE inhibitors, alcohol, analgesics, chloramphenicol, sulphanamides, quinolones, MAOI, antifungals, beta blockers, H2 blocks, uricosuric agents. Its concentrations are decreased in concomitant use of rifampicin and antipsychotics.

* Carbimazole is to be avoided in patients with obstruction of the trachea. It may cause agranulocytosis and alopecia.

* Furazolidone is **contraindicated** in infants below 1 month, primaquine sensitivity and is to be used with caution in patients with G-6-P-D deficiency, pregnancy, lactation and tyramine containing foods.

* Lactulose is contraindicated in galactosemia and intestinal obstruction.

* Desmopressin is used in oesophageal varices, diabetes insipidus, nocturnal enuresis, mild to moderate hemophilia, hemophilia type A, von Willebrand type I and is contraindicated in vascular disease, CAD, chr. nephritis and von Willebrand's type II B.

* Effects of desmopressin are increased by carbamazepine and chlorpropamide.

* Omeprazole and Cisapride is **contraindicated** in pregnancy and lactation.

* Sucralfate, an antacid and antiulcer agent is contraindicated in severe renal impairment .

* Glycerine is used in narrow angle glaucoma.

* Clonazepam is **contraindicated** in respiratory insufficiency.

* Mebendazole is **contraindicated** in children below two years and may cause alopecia and agranulocytosis.

* Cimetidine inhibits metabolism of mebendazole.

* Albendazole is **contraindicated** in pregnancy, children below 2 years and hepatic cirrhosis.

* Ketoconazole may cause gynaecomastia and oligospermia.

* Griseofulvin accelerates metabolism of oral contraceptives.

* Levodopa is **contraindicated** in melanoma and undiagnosed skin lesions.

* Pyridoxine, benzodiazepines and hydantoin reduces the effectiveness of Levodopa.

* Praziquantel is **contraindicated** in ocular cysticercosis.

* Dapsone is contraindicated in severe anemia and advanced renal amyloidosis.

* Ethambutol may cause joint pain and precipitation of gout.

* Streptomycin, in addition to TB, is used in infections by H. influenzae, Klebsiella pneumonia, E. coli, Proteus, Enterococcus faecalis and Str. Viridans.

* Griseofulvin is **contraindicated** in SLE.

* Antacids increase effectiveness of Levodopa.

* Heparin may cause throbocytopenia, alopecia, osteoporosis and hepatic dysfunction.
* Protamine may produce flushing.
* Dicyclomine, an antispasmodic is contraindicated in infants below 6 months and narrow angle glaucoma.
* Pharmacogenetics are important in metabolism of Isoniazid.
* **Maximum** enterohepatic circulation is seen in Ampicillin.
* With Tamoxifen, retinal pigmentation is a side effect.
* Drug unergoing Entero Hepatic circulation is Erythromycin.
* Loading dose of a drug is given when serum concentration is to be achieved rapidly.
* The maximum effect of a drug is defined as efficacy.
* Antiepileptic drug **contraindicated** in a child <3 yr is sodium valproate.
* Drug absorbed by active transport is levodopa.
* Nifedipine is to be avoided in angina.
* Drug which is not used in chronic CHF is dobutamine.
* Quinidine even in higher doses is not toxic because it goes intracellularly.
* Drug most effective in prinzmetal angina diltiazem.
* Non-ischaemic chest pain is caused by vincristine.
* **Most common** side effect of antihypertensive medication is depression.
* **Maximum effect** on the contractility of heart is seen with verapamil.
* Puinidine is contraindicated in Bifascicular block, thyrotoxicsis and acute carditis.
* Nimodipine is a Cerebro selective calcium channel-blocker.
* Magnesium sulphate potentiates the hypotensive action of methyl dopa.
* **K+ channel opener** is minoxidil.
* Maximum prolongation of ventricular repolarization is by Amiodarone.

* Ranitidine is 5 times more potent than cimetidine.

* Anti ulcer drug, not affected by food is cimetidine.

* Antiemetic contraindicated in pregnancy is metoclopramide.

* Paralytic ileus is caused by Cisplatinum.

* **Ondansterone** acts by 5-HT3 inhibition.

* Decreased gastric acid secretion is by PGE2.

* Diphenoxylate acts on receptors.

* Diuretic that acts only on PCT is Acetazolamide.

* Diuretic used in diabetes patients is Chlorthiazide.

* Renal excretion of drugs is not influenced by Lipid solubility.

* **Probenecid** decreases the urinary excretion of Cejuroxime, Cadotaxime, and Cefazolin.

* As compared to cyclopenthiazide, frusemide is less potent and more efficacious.

* **Hyperkalemia** may occur if potassium sparing diureties are given along with captopril or other ACE inhibitors.

* **In CRF**, Triamterene is contraindicated.

* Cirrhosis of liver is caused by Methotrexate.

* **Halofantrine** is used for resistant P. falciparum malaria.

* **Longest** acting bronchodilator is Bitolterol.

* The inducers of cyt. P450 are Phenytoin, Phenobarbitone and Rifampicin.

* Drug of choice in Theophylline poisoning is Propranolol.

* A drug, which lowers both HDL & LDL, given in hyperlipidemia is Probucol.

* Azithromycin is used as a superior drug to erythromycin in H. influenzae treatment.

* Concomitant administration of drug which enhances the CNS side effect of Ciprofloxacin is Doxycycline.

* Phototoxic rash is seen with Doxycycline.

* Bleeding due to excessive dosage of dicumarol is best treated by parenteral administration of Mnadione.

* Maximum reduction in level of plasma triglycerides is achieved by Nicotinamide.
* Oral anticoagulants cause craniofacial defect in fetus
* Buspirone acts on 5HT1a.
* Zidovidine acts by inhibiting the reverse transcriptase.
* Actinomycin D acts on Transcription.
* Best drug available for HIV infections is AZT.
* Local anesthetic antitussive is Benzonatate.
* Nocturnal leg cramps can be releaved by quinine.
* Pyrazinamide forms part of multi-drug regimen in tuberculosis because it kills ultracellular oganisms.
* **Ivermectin** is a Filaricide.
* Drug useful in chloroquine resistant malaria is mefloquine.
* Mefloquine should not be used with Verapamil.
* Antifungal drug causing renal toxicity is Amphotericin-B.
* Hyperuricemia, hyperglycemia and hypercalcemia are seen with Thiazide diuretics.
* Glucagon receptors are on cell membrane.
* Syndrome of inappropiate ADH secretion (**SIADH**) is caused by Chlorpropamide.
* Insulinoma is diagnosed by Tolbutamide.
* **Mifepristone** is used for termination of pregnancy.
* Estrogen treatment is associated with Hepatocellular adenoma.
* Endocrine manifestations as a side effect are caused by Ketoconazole.
* **Most common** side effect of prolonged use of steroids is affective disorders.
* Androgen, estrogen and progesterone act on protein regulation through nuclear receptor except GnRH.
* Galamine agents can produce tachycardia through an atropine like effect.
* Amiodarone does not cause hypokalaemia.

* Cholesterol levels are increased by Corticosteroids.
* Probucol is a cholesterol lowering agent that lowers cholesterol without any effect on triglyceride and dose is 500 mg b.d.
* Cartilage damage in children is caused by Quinolones.
* Hirsutism is seen with Minoxidil therapy.
* Spironolactone induced hyperkalemia is potentiated by beta blocker, Captopril, Nifedipine and NSAIDS.
* Clofazimine is an example of "dye".
* Rhabdomyolysis may be produced by aspirin.
* Sulfonamides may produce eosinophilia.
* Sulindac is a derivative of Indole.
* After stopping disulfiram, sensitization to alcohol lasts for 7-14 days.
* If a patient on oral corticosteroids is to be anaesthesized, give 100 mg hydrocortisone intraoperatively.
* Convulsions are complications of Cimetidine.
* Half life of Pefloxacin quinolone is maximum.
* Fentanyl-droperidol are usually used in fixed combination of 0.05, 2.5 mg respectively.
* Albendazole, Praziquantel and Pyrantel pamoate antiheiminthics are contraindicated in pregnancy except Piperazine.
* Adenosine has a very short half life due to uptake by epithelial cells and RBC's
* The class IV drug increases the ERP of bypass tract in heart is Verapamil.
* Treatment of choice in Wolf-Parkinson White syndrome is Cardioversion.
* Etoposide is an Anticancer drug.
* Alprostadil is used in neonates with congenital heart defects till surgery is undertaken.
* Misoprostol can be used in peptic ulcer.
* Erythromycin has to be given with caution with antiepileptic Carbamazepine.

* When given to a patient on phenytoin, dose of theophylline should be 1.5 times.

* 5-Aminosalicylic acid is useful in Ulcerative colitis.

* Levamisole is contrainidcated when ether or TCE anaesthesia is used

* Epoprostenol is a PG12 analogue.

* Doxorubicin is a DNA intercalator and generates free radicals.

* Etidronate sodium is best used in Paget's disease.

* Sparfloxacin is characterized by convulsions, hallucinations and cutaneous allergy.

* Pregnancy should be avoided upto 6 months even after withdrawal of gold therapy

* Ammoidine is used in Psoriasis.

* Most effective macrolide against chlamydia is Clarithromycin.

* Ftorafur is a anticancer drug.

* Lidoflazine is most useful in Angina.

* Rapid injection of analgin may produce Hypotension.

* Ergotamine is absolutely contraindicated in Roxithromycin therapy.

* Lisinopril is contraindicated in aortic stenosis.

* Pyrogallol causes COMP inhibition.

* Pergoilide has the of causes sideeffects of Retroperitoneal fibrosis, Hallucinosis and Erythromyalgia.

* Dose of selegiline higher than 10 mg may induce inhibition of MAO-A.

* Rash is most common sideffect of rifabutin.

* Main sideeffects of higher dose of clarithromycin is on hearing.

* Trientine is a useful alternative for Penicillamine.

* Adverse effects of propafenone therapy includes reentrant Vent. tachycardia, exacerbation of CHF and bronchospasm.

* Lamotrigine acts on Na+Channels.

* Succimer is a useful antidote for arsenic, mercury and cadmium and not Copper.

* Vigabatrin is useful for Mania.

* Dose of a drug for a child is obtained by multiplying the adult dose by the age of the child at his next birthday and dividing by 24 is Cowling rule.

* 'Drug-fast' is a term used for **drug Resistance.**

* A quantity of drug several times larger than the maintenance dose used as a initiation therpay to rapidly establish the desired blood and tissue levels of drug is **priming dose.**

* The side effects of ondansetronare headache, allergy and constipation.

* Moricizine, a phenothiazine analog is mainly used for the treatment of Ventricular arrythmias.

* Preventive treatment of recurrent episodes of **torsades de points** is **magnesium sulphate**.

* Propafenone is mainly a Na+ channel blocker.

* **Surrogate marker** is a clinical or lab test that correlates with clinical outcome of a disease.

* Lipid soluble nonionized drugs most easily cross placental barrier.

* **Pergolide** is mainly used for Parkinsonism.

* Insulin resistance is transmitted by IgG.

* Warfarin which may be given I/V is Warfarin sodium.

* **Most potent oestrogen** is Estradiol.

* Drugs which **inhibit spermatogenesis** are danazol, ethinyl oestradiol and proxypropione.

* Neutropenia is a sideeffects of Ticlodipine.

* Headache, Diarrhoea or constipation are side effects of granisetron.

* Rifabutin acts on **RNA polymerase.**

* Drug fever, skin rash and neutropenia are sideeffects of Teicoplanin.

* Gabapentin causesataxia, somnolence and fatigue.

* Homatropine is a combination of Mandelicacid + tropine.

* Main indication of **olanzepine** is Schizophrenia.

* **Skin blush** or flush may be produced by Atropine.
* **Baclofen** acts on K^+ and Ca^{++} ions conductance but not on Na^+.
* **Bretazenil** is useful in Panic attacks.
* **Tacrine** has been tried in Alzhiemer's disease.
* **Natamycin** is useful for fungal blephritis.
* **Polygeline** is a plasma volume substitute.
* **Nicorandil** mainly acts on K+Channel.
* Rivavirin is used with caution in Asthma, Hypertension and Anemia.
* Following interact with perindopril—Cyclosporine —> hyperkalemia, OCP —>antagonise hypotensive effect and Alcohol —> Enhanced hypotension.

TREATMENT/DRUG OF CHOICE (DOC)

* Anoxic spells of TOF—**Morphine**
* Prophylaxis of anoxic spells of TOF—**Propranolol**
* Acute attack of angina—**Nitroglycerin**
* Ventricular tachycardia—**Lidocaine (Xylocaine)**

Ventricular Fibrillation and Flutter :

* Treatment of choice—**Defibrillation**
* Drug of choice—**Bretylium**

  (external cardiac massage and prompt ventilation until electric defibrillation is available)
* Digitalis induced ventricular arrhythmias —**Lidocaine and phenytoin**
* Stokes-Adams attack with heart block—**Isoprenaline**
* Dressler's syndrome—**Indomethacin or corticosteroids**
* Sinus bradycardia (55/mt) —**Ephedrine or atropine**
* Paroxysmal atrial tachycardia (170-220/mt)—**Verapamil**
* Atrial fibrillation (400-600/mt)—**Digitalis**
* Atrial flutter (250-350/mt)—**Digitalis** (if counter shock is not available)

* Ventricular premature beats — **Lidocaine**
* Paroxysmal ventricular tachycardia (160-240/mt)—**DC counter shock (DOC: Lidocaine)**
* Sinoatrial block—**No treatment/atropine**
* Ventricular prexcitation (WPW syndrome) with atrial fibillation—**DC cardioversion**
* Primary pulmonary hypertension—**Oral phentolamine**
* DOC in emergency management of acute asthama—**Epinephrine and IV aminophylline**
* States asthmaticus or acute attacks in epinephrine resistant patients—**IV hydrocortisone and methyl prednisolone (preparation of choice)**
* DOC in Klebsiella pneumonia is **Cephalothin (alternative Gentamicin)**
* Streptococcal pneumonia—**Penicillin G**
* DOC in Legionella pneumonia **Erythromicin**
* DOC in pneumocystitis carinii pneumonia is **Sulfamethoxazole-trimethoprim (alternative pentamidine isothionate)**
* Lung abscess—**postural drainage and bronchoscopy (initial drug : Penicillin)**
* Pulmonary embolism—**Adequate prolongation of the clotting time with heparin** (treatment of choice)
* H. influenza pneumonia—**Ampicillin**
* DOC in carcinoid lung is **Doxorubicin**
* Large cell ca. lung—**Surgery**
* Small cells (oat cell) ca. lung—**combination chemotherapy**
* Diverticulitis—**Ampicillin**
* Whipple's disease—**Tetracycline**
* Tropical sprue—**Tetracycline**
* Carcinoid syndrome with secondaries in liver—**5 Flurouracil** into the hepatic artery
* Carcinoid syndrome with repeated flushes—**Prednisolone**
* Strawberry lesion of rectosigmoid—**Acetarsol suppository with vitamin C**

* Urinary analgesic—**Phenozopyridine**
* Nocturnal eneuresis—**Imipramine**
* Antibiotics safe in renal failure with modified dosage
  — **Penicillin**
  — **Vancomycin**
  — **Gentamicin**
  — **Cephalothin**
* Septicaemia from pyelonephritis—**Gentamicin**

Calcium Stones :

* Idiopathic hypercalciuria—**Thiazide diuretics**
* Hyperuricosuria—**Allopurinol or diet**
* Primary hyperparathyroidism—**Surgery**
  Distal renal tubular acidosis—**Alkali replacement**
* Intestinal hyperoxaluria—**Cholestyramine or oral calcium loading**
* Hereditary hyperoxaluria—**Fluids and pyridoxine**
* Idiopathic stone disease—**Oral phosphates, fluids**

Uric Acid Stones :

* Gout—**Alkali to raise urine pH**
* Idiopathic—**Allopurinol** (if daily urine uric acid is 1000 mg)
* Dehydration—**Alkalifluids, reversal of cause**
* Lesch-Nyhan syndrome—**Allopurinol**
* Malignant tumours—**Allopurinol**
* Cystine stones—**Massive fluids, Alkali D-pencillamine**
* Struvite stones—**Antimicrobial agents and Judicious surgery**
* Bladder bacteriuria (Cystitis)—**Single dose of IM 500 mg Kannamycin**
* Acute uncomplicated cystitis (90% due to E. coli)—**Co-trimoxazole single dose**
* Acute urethritis (in women chlamydial infection)—**Doxycycline 100 mg bid/7 dyas**
* Acute pyelonephritis—**Co-trimoxazole 10-14 days**

* Acute cystitis (in pregnancy)—**Amoxicillin 7 days**
* Prophylactic UTI—**Co-trimoxazole (single dose)**
* Symptomatic infections—**Nitrofurantoin 50-100 mg (after sexual intercourse)**
* Diabetes insipidus—**Vasopressin, Desmopressin (DDAVP)**
* Thyrotoxicosis patients preparing for thyroidectomy—**Propylthiouracil and Iodine (preopmethod of choice)**
* Thyrotoxicosis in pregnancy—**Propranolol**
* Hypoparathyroid testing—calciferol
* Adrenal crisis—**Hydrocortisone sodium succinate.**
* Addison's disease—**Hydrocortisone**
* Hypercalcemia due to hypervitaminosis D—**Steroids**
* Autoimmune haemolytic anemia—**Prednisone** (initial TOC) but when corticosteroids fail —splenectomy to be considered
* ALL (Acute lymphatic leukaemia)—**Multiple drug therapy**
— Vincristine arrests cell in mitosis, prednisone lyses lymphoblasts in resting phase, or prevents their entry into DNA synthesis, mercaptopurine inhibits DNA synthesis, methotrexate inhibits DNA, RNA and protein synthesis.

Others : L-asparaginase, Daunorubicin, Etoposide and cytosine arabinoside

AML (acute myeloid leukaemia)—**Daunorubicin, cytosine arabinoside, Etoposide and thioguanine**
* CML—**Busulphanand hydroxyurea**
* CLL—**Chlorambucil**
* CLL in laterstages—**CHOP** (Cyclophosphamide, Doxorubicin, vincristine and Prednisolone)
* **Hodgkin's Lymphoma—Chemotherapy is indicated in**
    * All patients with 'B' symptoms
    * Stage II (with 3 years of involvement)
    * Stage III and IV

* CHL VPP regimen

  (Chlorambucil, Vinblastine, procarbazine and Prednisolone)

  Note : (Chlorambucil replaces, mustine in previous MOPP/MVPP regimen)

* **Non Hodgkin's Lymphoma**

  Stage I and II A — Involved field radiotherapy

  Stage II B and III — Chemotherapy

  Stage II — Whole body irradiation

* Burkitt's myeloma—**Aggressive therapy regimen :** Adriamycin + BCNV + cyclophosphamide + Melphalan

* Waldenstrom's macroglobulinaemia—**Chlorambucil**

* von Willebrand disease—**cryoprecipitate** (plasma fraction enriched in vWF)

* Haemophilia A — **Factor VIII concentrate**

* Christmas disease—**Factor IX concentrate**

* Reversal of warfarin for emergency surgery or overdose— **Vitamin K.**

* Reversal of heparin—**Protamine sulphate**

CONTRAINDICATION

---

* H/o previus mental depression—**Reserpine**

* MAOI with combination of any **antihypertensive drugs**

* Acute rheumatic fever associated with cardiac failure—**Sodium salicylate or sodium bicarbonate**

* AMI—**Second dose of morphine** if resp. are below 12/min.

* AF occurs in W-P-W syndrome—**Digitalis**

* Ventricular tachycardia—**Digitalis**

* Left ventricular failure—**Beta-adrenergic blocking drugs (propranolol)**

* ASD with pulmonary hypertension and shunt reversal—**Surgery**

* Hypertrophic cardiomyopathy and AV conduction blocks— **Digoxin**

* Sinus tachycardia or Digitalis toxicity—**Cardioversion**
* A non-glycoside positive ionotropic drug with associated vasodilator effect—**Amrinone**
* Chronic obstructive pulmonary disease—**Cough suppressing drugs**
* Asthmatic patients with hypertension or angina or in elderly patients —**Epinephrine**
* Severe asthma—**Sedation**
* Haemoptysis in pulmonary TB—**Morphine**
* Lumbar puncture—**Posterior fossa tumours**
* Ergotamine—**Septic or infectious hypertensive heart disease and pregnant women**
* Barbiturates—**Parkinsonism**
* High carbohydrate foods—**Familial periodic paralysis.**
* In an unconscious patient to keep airways upon the head should be well extended never **supine nor headflexed**
* Give 100 mg thiamine chloride IV before glucose in alcoholics to avert potentiation of Wernicke's encephalopathy by glucose
* **Iron-sorbitol** should be given by intramuscular injection, never intravenously.
* **Iron-dextran** is seldom given intramuscularly but can be given intravenously by 'total dose infusion method'
* **G6 PD deficiency**—avoid antimalarials and sulphonamides.
* **Pyronaridine** is an antimalarial drug.
* **Therapeutic window phenomenon:** Optimal therapeutic effect is exerted over a narrow range of plasma concentrations or drug doses; both below and above the range, beneficial effects are suboptimal. e.g : Nortriptytine (tricyclic antidepresant), clonidine, glipizide etc.

GENERAL PHARMACOLOGY

THE PLASMA PROTEIN BINDING OF CERTAIN DRUGS

Penicillins :

Ampicillin	25%
Methicillin	40%
Benzylpenicillin	60%
Phenoxymethylpenicillin	80%
Cloxacillin	95%

The sulphonamides :

Sulphadimidine	30% (rapidly excreted)
Sulphadiazine	50% (rapidly excreted)
Sulphamethoxypyridazine	85% (slowly excreted)
Sulphadimethoxine	95% (slowly excreted)

The barbiturates :

Barbitone	5%
Phenobarbitone	20%
Pentobarbitone	37%
Thiopentone	65%

Some other examples of plasma protein binding :

Salicylate	50 to 80%
Warfarin	95%
Phenylbutazone	98%
Indomethacin	90%
Pethidine	40%

NEW DRUG DELIVERY SYSTEMS

(i)   **Ocusert** when placed directly under the eyelid can deliver a steady flow of pilocarpine round the clock for 7 days without causing any discomfort, thus avoiding the need for repeated eye drops.

(ii) **Progestasert** an intraulcerine contraceptive device, produces controlled release of minute quantities of progesterone within the uterus for a year.

(iii) **Prodrug** is an inactive chemical derivative that after administration, undergoes biotransformation to the pharmacologically active drug eg.

— Propoxyphene napsylate : propoxyphene.

DRUGS WITH A LOW THERAPEUTIC RATIO

(Effective dose close to toxic dose)	Procainamide
Aminoglycoside antibiotics	Propranolol
Amikacin	Disopyramide
Gentamicin	Quinidine
Kanamycin	Some antihypertensives
Tobramycin	*Antidepressants*
Netilmycin	Amitriptyline
Anticonvulsants/antiepileptics	Imipramine
Phenytoin	Nortriptyline
Barbiturates, e.g.phenobarbitone	Dothiepin
Primidone	Central nervous system depressants
Ethosuximide	Oral hypoglycaemic agents, e.g. sulphonylureas
Sodium Valproate	Warfarin and other anti-vitamin K oral anticoagulants
Carbamazepine	
Clonazepam	Theophylline, aminophylline
Cardiovascular system	Lithium preparations
Digoxin and digitalis glycosides	Methotrexate
Lignocaine	

BIOAVAILABILITY OF DRUG

Depends on
      tablet disintegration
      dissolution time
      excipients in tablet
      gut lumen pH
      gastric emptying time
      intestinal transit time
      gut surface area
      gut bacteria acting on drug
      state of gut
      surface area
      presence of disease process
      mesenteric blood flow
      first pass effect
These factors effect
      peak plasma concentration of drug after one dose time of
peak value

FACTORS AFFECTING CONCENTRATION OF A DRUG OR CHEMICAL IN THE BLOOD

Drug
      dosage
      use and dose
      route of administration
      concentration of toxic agent
      duration of exposure to the substance
Body factors
      age
      body weight
      time of sampling, related to time of dose
      presence of other drugs
      disease state
      of liver
      of kidney
      of other organs
      body water status
      menstruation
      any anatomical abnormalities
      any genetic abnormalities

Estimation

    time of sampling, and duration between sampling and estimation

    mode of storage of sample prior to estimation

Other factors

    gastrointestinal absorption rate

    tissue binding at active and inactive sites rate of elimination and inactivation

        storage

        bone

        hair

        nails

        fat

induction or inhibition of microsomal enzymes syner gism or antagonism by other drugs tolerance (prolonged use of drugs or drugs with cross-tolerance) addictive drug effects

Other side-effects

interference with absorption of other substances from the gastrointestinal tract

interference with immunity systems

interference with platelet function

DRUG INHIBITING DRUG METABOLISM

    Allopurinol

    Chloramphenicol

    Disulfiram

    Isoniazid

    Levodopa and methyldopa

    Hydrazine

    Methandrostenolone

    Monoamine oxidase inhibitors

    Nortriptyline

    Oral contraceptives

    Oxyphenylbutazone and phenylbutazone

    Para-aminosalicylate

    Perphenazine

    Phenyramidol

    Sulphaphenazole

    Sulthiame

FACTORS DETERMINING RATE OF ABSORPTION OF DRUGS

1. *Solubility :* soluble drus are quickly absorbed.

2. *Physical state :* colloids are slowy absorbed while crystalloids are quickly absorbed.

3. *Ionisation :* greater the ionisation slower is absorption.

4. *pH :* gastric pH 8 increases absorption of basic drugs.

5. *Surface area :* greater the absorbing surface quicker is the absorption

6. *Vascularity :* greater vascularity quicker absorption.

7. *Presence of another drug :* AI $(OH)_3$ gel retards absorption of many drugs (eg. Tetracycline).

DRUGS EXCRETED UNCHANGED BY THE KIDNEY

1. β-*blockers*—atenolol.

2. *Antibiotics*—penicillins; cephalosporins, aminoglyco-sides, tetracycline.

3. *Diuretics*—frusemide, chlorothiazide.

4. *Cardiac drugs*—digoxin, procainamide.

5. *CNS drugs*—lithium.

6. *Oral hypoglycaemics*—chlorpropamide, metformin.

7. *Analgesics*—aspirin (in overdosage only).

8. *Others*—cimetidine, ranitidine, gallamine

RECEPTORS INVOLVED IN DRUG ACTION

1. *Endorphin receptors*
   (a) Agonist—morphine
   (b) Antagonist—naloxone.
2. *Aldosterone receptors*
   Antagonists—spironolactone.
3. *Histamine receptors*
   (a) H_1 antagonists—chlorpheniramine, promethazine, terfenadine etc.
   (b) H_2 antagonists—cimetidine, ranitidine, famotidine.

4. *Dopamine (CNS) receptors*
   (a) Agonists—bromoergocriptine.
   (b) Antagonist—chlorpromazine.
5. α_1-*adrenergic (postsynaptic) receptors*
   Agonist—dopadine
6. α_2-adrenergic (brain stem) receptors
   Agonist—clonidine
7. β_1-*adrenergic receptors*
   (a) Agonist—dopamine.
   (b) Antagonist—metoprolol, atenolol.
8. $\beta 2$-adrenergic receptors
   Agonist — salbutanol

DRUGS UNDERGOING MAJOR HEPATIC METABOLISM

1. β-blockers—Propranolol, labetalol, metoprolol, oxprenolol.
   β_2-agonists—Salbutamol, terbutaline.
2. *Antibiotics*—Rifampicin, erythromycin.
3. *Diuretics*—Spironolactone.
4. *CNS drugs*—Chlormethiazole, tricyclics, phenothiazines, benzodiazepines barbiturates, L-DOPA.
5. *Cardiac drugs*—Glyceryl trinitrate, verapamil, nifedipine, lignocaine, prazosin, digitoxin.
6. *Oral hypoglycaemics*—Glibenclamide, tolbutamide
7. *Analgesics*—Paracetamol, pethidine, pentazocine, propoxyphene, aspirin.

EFFECT OF DRUGS ON NUTRIENT ABSORPTION AND METABOLISM

Drug	Effect
Analgesics and anti-inflammatories	
Salicylates	Decreases serum ascorbic acid; increases urinary loss of ascorbic acid, potassium, and amino acids.
Sulfasalazine	Impairs folate absorption and antagonizes folate supplementation

Antacids

Aluminium antacids	Decrease absorption of phosphate and vitamin A
Others	Alkaline destruction of thiamine; some decrease in absorption of vitamin A. iron; steatorrhoea

Anticonvulsants

Phenobarbital	Decreases serum folate; increases vitamin D and vitamin K turnover and may cause deficiency.
Phenytoin	Decreases serum folate; increases vitamin D and vitamin K turnover and may cause deficiency.
Primidone	Decreases serum folate and vitamins B6, B12, decreases calcium absorption, increases vitamin D and vitamin K turnover and may cause deficiency

Antimicrobials

Neomycin	Binds bile acids and decreased absorption of fat. carotene; vitamin A,D, K,B12 potassium, sodium, calcium nitrogen
Amphotericin B	Decreases serum magnesium and · potassium
Aminosalicyclic acid	Increases absorption of folate, vitamin B12, iron, cholesterol, fat
Chloramphenicol	Increases need for vitamin B2, B6, B12, increases serum iron.
Penicillin	Hypokalemia; renal potassium wasting
Tetracycline	Calcium, iron, magnesium inhibit drug absorption, decreases vitaminK synthetsis.
Cycloserine	May decrease absorption of calcium, magnesium; may decrease serum folate and vitamins B6, B12, decreases protein synthesis.

Isoniazid	Vitamin B6 antagonist; may cause deficiency.
Sulfonamides	Decrease absorption of folate; decrease serum folate, iron.
Nitrofurantoin	Decreases serum folate
Pyrimethamine	Decreases serum B12 and folate.

Antimitotics

| Methotrexate | Decreases absorption of folate, vitamin B12 and fat |
| Colchicine | Decreases absorption of vitamin B12, carotene, fat, sodium, potassium, cholesterol, lactose, nitrogen. |

Cathartics

| Phenolphthalein | Malabsorption hypokalemia; deficiency of vitamin D, calcium |
| Mineral oil | Malabsorption; decreased absorption of vitamins A,D,K. |

| **Diuretics** | Some cause hypokalemia, hypomagnesemia, may increase urinary excretion of vitamins B1, B6 calcium magnesium, potassium |

Hypocholesterolemics

| Cholestyramine | Binds bile acids; decreases absorption of fat, carotene, vitamins A,D,K,B12 folate, iron. |
| Clofibrate | Decreases absorption of carotene, vitamin B12, iron glucose |

Hypotensives

| Hydralazine | Vitamin B6 deficiency |
| Captopril | May cause hyponatremia, hyperkalemia; decreased taste acuity |

| **Oral contraceptives** | Vitamin B6, folate deficiency; may increase the need for other mutrients |

DRUG METABOLISM BY HEPATIC MICROSOMAL ENZYMES

* **Drugs commonly inhibiting cytochrome P450**

1. *Acute alcoholic binge.*
2. *Antibiotics*
   - (a) INH
   - (b) Erythromycin
   - (c) Sulphonamides
   - (d) Metronidazole
   - (e) Chloramphenicol
3. *Anticonvulsants*
   —Sodium valproate
4. *Other drugs*
   - (a) Cimetidine
   - (b) Allopurinol
   - (c) Chlorpromazine, imipramine
   - (d) Propranolol, metoprolol
   - (e) Dextropropoxyphene
   - (f) Disulfiram

* **Drugs commonly inducing cytochrome P450**

1. *Chronic alcohol ingestion or cigarette smoking*
2. *Antibiotics — rifampicin griseofulvin, Doxycycline*
3. *Anticonvulsants*
   - (a) Phenytoin
   - (b) Carbamazepine
   - (c) Phenobarbitone, primidone
4. *Analgesics*
   - (a) Phenylbutozone
   - (b) Antipyrene
5. *Hypnotics*
   - (a) Barbiturates
   - (b) Chloral hydrate
   - (c) Glutethionide
6. *Hypolipodemics*
   - (a) Clofibrate
   - (b) Halofenate
7. *Others*
   - (a) Aminoglutethimide
   - (b) Spironolactone
   - (c) Griseofulvin
   - (d) Ethanol
   - (e) Lindane, DDT

DIET INDICATIONS

Diet indicated in High Quantities :

Fiber :
* Diverticulitis
* Irritable bowel syndrome

Proteins and Calories :
* PEM

Calcium :
* Osteoporosis

Potassium :
* Diuretic therapy

DIET CONTRAINDICATIONS

Diet Completely restricted in :

Sodium : is contraindicated in :
* Hypertension
* Congestive heart failure
* Chronic liver disease
* Chronic renal failure

Potassium—Chronic renal failure

Copper—Wilson's disease

Phosphate—Chronic renal failure

Aminoacid—Phenylketonuria

Tyramine—Monoamine oxidase inhibitor use

Protein—Hepatic encephalopathy

—Chronic renal failure

Calorie —Obesity
—Diabetes (type II)

Fat—Malabsorption syndromes

Fat and Cholesterol—Hyperlipidemia
—Diabetes mellitus

Lactose—Lactose intolerance

Gluten—Coeliac sprue

Oxalate—Hyperoxaluria

Salicylate—Chronic urticaria

Diet elimination—Food allergies

DRUG INCOMPATIBILITIES IN INTRAVENOUS FLUIDS

Drug	Incompatible with	Reason
The Penicillins	Tetracyclines (HCl)	Precipitation
	Gentamicin	Inactivation of Gentamicin
Carbenicillin	Kanamycin	Inactivation of Carbenicillin
	Colistin	Inactivation of Colistin
	Gentamicin	Inactivation of Gentamicin
Tetracyclines	Penicillin	Precipitation

(HCl)	Sulfonamide (Na+ Salts)	Precipitation
	Hydrocortisone Sodium Succinate	Precipitation
	Calcium Salts	Tetracycline chelate formed
	Cephaloridine	Precipitation
	Sodium Bicarbonate	Precipitation
Heparin Sodium	Hydrocortisone Sodium Succinate	Precipitation
	Sympathomimetic amines	Precipitation
	Tetracyclines	Precipitation
	Aminoglycoside Antibiotics	Precipitation
	(Gentamicin, Kanamycin, Streptomycin)	

THERAPEUTIC RANGE OF VARIOUS COMMONLY USED DRUGS

Drug	Serum therapeutic	Range
Digoxin	1.0-ng/ml	1.3-2.6 nmol/L
Ethosuximide	30-100µg/ml	210-710 µmol/L
Phenobarbtone	10-30 µg/ml	40-130 µmol/L
Phenytoin	10-20 µg/ml	40-80 µmol/L
Primidone	5-15 µg/ml	25-70 µmol/L
Carbamazepine	3-9 µg/ml	13-38 µmol/L
Diazepam	400-500 ng/m*	—
Valproate	50-100 µg/ml	350-700 µmol/L
Theophylline	10-20 µg/ml	—
Lithium	0.6-1.2 meq/L	0.4-1.5 meq/L

* Anticonvulsant dose

PRESCRIBING DRUGS IN HEPATIC DISEASE

Reduced dose necessary	* Lignocaine (metabolism impaired)
	* Paracetamol (dose causing hepatotoxicity reduced)
	* Phenytoin (metabolism impaired)
	* Propranolol (metabolism impaired)
	* ?Propranolol (metabolism impaired, not other beta blockers)
	* Rifampicin (biliary excretion impaired)
	* Thiopentone (protein binding impaired)

Avoid

* Antacids causing constipation (ppt. encephalopathy)
* Antidepressants (ppt. encephalopathy)
* Aspirin (risk of G.I. bleeding)
* Biguanides (may cause lactic acidosis)
* Diuretics (thiazides and loop diuretics —> hypokalemia may ppt encephalopathy)
* Erythromycin (cholestatic jaundice)
* Lomotil (ppt. encephalopathy)
* Opiates (ppt. encephalopathy)
* Phenylbutazones (fluid retention)
* Phenothiazines (ppt. encephalopathy)
* Sedative (ppt. encephalopathy)
* Sulfonylureas (may cause cholestatic jaundice)
* Tetracyclines (i.v. doses > 1 g daily hepatotoxic)
* Warfarin — decreased synthesis of clotting factors)

DRUGS EXHIBITING SATURATION KINETICS

1. Phenytoin.
2. Salicylate
3. Alcohol

DISEASES ASSOCIATED WITH SLOW ACETYLATION PHENOTYPE

1. Gilbert's syndrome
3. Arylamine-induced bladder cancer.
2. Sjogren's syndrome.

RATIONALE FOR DETERMINING THE ACETYLATION PHENOTYPE

(50% of the population are slow acetylators)

1. **Isoniazid.**

   (a) *Slow acetylators*

       (i)   ↑ Peripheral neuropathy (B6)

       (ii)   ↑ Iatrogenic SLE

       (iii) ↑ Phenytoin/carbamazepine toxicity.

       (iv) ↑ Rifampicin-induced hepatotoxicity.

   (b) *Rapid acetylators*

       (i)   ↑ Failure or once-wkly TB therapy

       (ii)   ↑ INH-induced hepatitis.

2. **Sulphasalazine** (slow acetylators)

   (a) ↑ Toxicity from sulphapyridine moiety, especially **headaches,** leucopenia,

   (b) ↑ Haemolysis in G6PD-deficient patients

3. **Hydralazine**

   (a) *Slow acetylators*—Iatrogenic SLE, especially in females

   (b) *Rapid acetylators*—Failure of antihypertensive therapy.

4. **Procainamide**—Slow acetylators : iatrogenic SLE.

5. **Dapsone**

   (a) *Slow acetylators*—Haemolysis in G6PD deficient patients.

   (b) *Rapid acetylators*—Failure of therapy for dermatitis herpetiformis.

MECHANISMS OF DRUG INTERACTIONS

	Mechanisms	Example	Effect
1.	Pharmaceutical incompatibility	Thiopentone and suxamethonium	Precipitate
2.	Interference with drug absorption	Opioid analgesics and orally administered drugs	Delayed absorption
3.	Changes in drug distribution	Aspirin and warfarin	Bleeding
4.	Change in hepatic metabolism		
	a) enzyme induction	Phenobarbitone and warfarin	Reduced effect of warfarin
	b) enzyme inhibition	Cimetidine and many other drugss	Prolonged effect
	c) changes in liver blood flow	Halothane and ketamine	Delayed elimination of keta-mine
6.	Interference with excretion		
	a) renal	Probenecid and penicillin	High penicillin concentration
	b) biliary	—	—
7.	Antagonism or potentiation by drugs acting on the same physiological system or at the same time.	Alcohol and barbiturates	Potentiation
8.	Change in fluid and electrolyte balance	Diuretics and digoxin	Digoxin toxicity
9.	Miscellaneous		
	a) monoamine oxidase inhibition	MAOI and tyramine	Hypertensive crisis
	b) antagonism of antibiotics	—	—

CVS

CLASSIFICATION OF BETA ADRENERGIC BLOCKING AGENTS

	Drug	Partial agonist effect (intrinsic sympathomimetic effect)	Membrane stabilising effect (quinidine like effect)
Division I : non-selective ($\beta_1+\beta_2$) block			
Group I	Oxprenolol Alprenolol	+	+
Group II	Propranolol	−	+
Group III	Pindolol	+	−
Group IV	Sotalol Timolol Nadolol	−	−
Division II : cardioselective block (β_1)*			
Group I	Acebutolol	+	+
Group III	Practolol Atenolol	+	−
Group IV	Metoprolol	−	−
Division III : non-selective block + alpha - block			
Group II	Labetalol	−	+
Division IV : cardioselective block + alpha-block			
	no example yet available.		

IMPORTANT CARDIAC GLYCOSIDES

Source	Precursor Glycosides	Glycoside	Sugar	Aglycone or Genin
Digitalis purpurea (leaf)	Purpurea Glycoside A (desacetyl-digilanid A)	Digitoxin	Digitoxose	Digotoxigenin
	Purpurea Glycoside B (desacetyl-digilanid B)	Gitoxin	Digitoxose	Gitoxigenin
	—	Gitalin	Digitoxose	Gitaligenin
	Lanatoside A (digilanid A)	Digitoxin	Digitoxose	Digitoxigenin
Digitalis lanata (leaf)	Lanatoside B (digilanid B)	Gitoxin	Digitoxose	Gitoxigenin
	Lanatoside C (digilanid C Cedialanid)	Digoxin	Digitoxose	Digoxigenin

DOSE OF ORAL DIGOXIN

Age	Total digitalizing dose (mg/kg)	Daily maintenance dose (mg/kg)
Under 1 month	0.04	0.01
1—18 months	0.08	0.02
18 months—6 years	0.06	0.015
6—12 years	0.04	0.01

PHARMACOKINETICS OF ORAL DIGOXIN AND DIGITOXIN

	Digoxin	Digitoxin
Absorption	60-85%	90-100%
Plasma protein binding	Minimal	Extensive
Disposal	70% metabolized, 30% excreted unchanged	Metabolized completely
Enterohepatic recycling	6-8 %	Extensive
Plasma half life effect after stopping	24-48 hours	5 days
Time for digitalization without loading dose	5-7 days	25-30 days
Time for effect of a single dose	4-6 hours	6-8 hours
Persistence of effect after stopping.	3-6 days	18 days

CONTRAINDICATIONS TO DIGITALIS THERAPY

1. The only absolute contraindication is digitalis toxicity
2. Recent myocardial infarction
3. Partial or complete heart block
4. Stokes Adams syndrome.
5. W.P.W. syndrome.
6. Diphtheritic myocarditis
7. Constrictive pericarditis
8. Ventricular tachycardia.
9. Pressence of tight M.S.
10. Grossly damaged myocardium.

EFFECTS OF DIGITALIS IN CCF

* ↑ in cardiac output & venous return.
* ↑ in stroke volume.
* ↓ in venous pressure
* / in diastolic heart size
* ↓ in heart rate
* Disappearance of oedema
* Diuresis
* B.P. Settles

INTERACTIONS OF DIGOXIN

* **↑ Digoxin toxicity/effect**

Diuretics (K+ losing)

Ca++

Quinidine

Verapamil

Dittiazem

Amiodarone

K+ sparing diuretics (*de renal excretion)

Adrenergic drugs

Succinylcholine

* **↓ Digoxin absorption**

Metoclopramide

Sucralfate

Antacids

* **↑ Digoxin absorption**

Atropinic drugs

(atropine, TCA's)

* **↑ Digoxin metabolism**

Phenobarb

USE OF I.V. ANTIARRHTHMIC AGENTS (IN ORDER OF PRIORITY) IN SUPRA VENTRICULAR ARRYTHMIAS

Sinus Tachycardia :
Propranolol—Verapamil
Atrial Tachyarrhthmias :
Verapamil—Propranolol—Procainamide—Quinidine
Nodal Tachycardia :
Propranolol—Verapamil—Procainamide
W P W Syndrome with Tachycardia :
Procainamide—Lidocaine—Verapamil—Propranolol

VENTRICULAR ARRHTHMIAS

Ventricular Premature Beats
Lidocaine—>Procainamide—>Propranolol—>Bretylium
Ventricular T chycardia
Lidocaine—>Procainamide—>Propranolol—>Bretylium
Ventricular Fibrillation
Bretylium

CLINICAL CLASSIFICATION OF CALCIUM ANTAGONISTS

Group I : Agents that block voltage - dependent Ca^{++} channels in myocardium and arteries.

(a)   No action on SA or AV nodes; No E.P. effects.

— *Dihydropyridines :* nifedipine, nicardipine, niludipine, nimodipine, nisoldipine, nitrendipine, ryosidine.

(b)   Additional action on SA and AV nodes : E.P. effects.

— *Phenylalkylamines :* verapamil, gallopamil, anipamil.

— *Benzothiazepines:* diltiazem

GROUP II : Block Ca^2+ channels in the muscle of arteries but spare the myocardium

— Diphenylpiperazines : cinnarizine, flunarizine.

GROUP III*   Action on Ca^{2+} and fast $Na+$ channels and have selective E.P. effects :

— bencyclane, bepridil, caroverine, etafenone, fendiline, lidoflazine, perhexiline, prenylamine, tiapamil

* = most of group withdrawn

E.P.   =   electrophysiologic

AV   =   atrioventricular

SA   =   Sinoatrial

CLINICAL INDICATIONS FOR BETA-BLOCKERS (CARDIOVASCULAR)

1. Angina pectoris

2. Hypertension

3. Arrhythmias

4. Recurrent ventricular fibrillation

5. Prevention of cardiac death in the postmyocardial infarction patient

6. Reduction in size and incidence of myocardial infarction

7. Dissecting aneurysm

8. Hypertrophic cardiomyopathy

9. Mitral valve prolapse syndrome

10. Q-T prolongation syndromes

11. Hypertensive response to endotracheal intubation

12. Tetralogy of Fallot

CLINICAL INDICATIONS FOR BETA-BLOCKERS (NON-CARDIAC)

1. Glaucoma

2. Migraine

3. Thyrotoxicosis

4. Anxiety and essential tremor

5. Delirium tremens and tetanus

6. Narcotic withdrawal and cocaine toxicity

7. Narcolepsy

8. Insulinoma

9. Bartter's syndrome (juxtaglomerular hyperplasia)

PRINCIPAL EFFECTS OF ANTIARRHYTHMIC DRUGS ON THE HEART

	Group I (Quinidine, Procainamide, Disopyramide)	Group II (Lignocaine, Phenytoin)	Group III (Propranolol)	Group IV (Verapamil)
Electrophysiological				
Automaticity	Decrease	Decrease	Decrease	Decrease
Excitability	Decrease	No change	Decrease	Decrease
Conduction velocity	Decrease or increase	No change	Decrease	Decrease
Electrocardiogram				
P-R duration	No change or increase	No change or decrease	No change or increase	No change or increase
QRS duration	Increase	No change	No change	No change
Q-T duration	Increase or decrease	No change or decrease	No change	No change
Hemodynamic				
Blood pressure	No change or decrease	No change or decrease	No change or decrease	No change or decrease
Cardiac output	Decrease	No change or decrease	Decrease	Decrease
Contractility	Decrease	No change or decrease	Decrease	Decrease
Left ventricular end diastolic pressure	May increase	No change or increase	May increase	May increase

PHARMACOLOGY OF NEW ANTIARRYTHMIC DRUGS

Drug	Protein binding (%)	t12 (h)	Effective concentration (mg/L)	Bioavailability (% dose) drugs	Excretion of uncharged (%)
Mexiletine	50-60	8-12	0.75-2.0	90	20
Tocainide	50	12-16	3-9	90	30-50
Flecainide	40	14-18	0.2-1.0	95	25
Encainide	90	2-3	0.5-3.0	80-90	10
Propafenone	95	6	0.5-3.0	80-90	<5
Amiodarone		10-50 days	1-2	50	
Sotalol	0	6-8	4	>90	>90
Pirmenol	80	4-17	1.0	80-90	50
Cibenzoline	60	4	0.2-0.4	90	>50
Ethmozine		5	0.5-1.0	80	

ELECTROPHYSIOLOGICAL EFFECTS OF SOME NEW ANTIARRYTHMIC DRUGS

Drug	SNRT	Conduction interval		Refractory periods			
		AH	HV	QRS	QT	HP	Ventricular
Mixiletine		↓/–			→		↓/–
Tocainide		↓/–			→		↓
Flecainide	↑	↑	↑	↑/–	↑	↑	↑
Encainide	↑/–		↑	↑	↑/–	↑/–	↑/–
Propafenone	↑	↑	↑/–	↑			↑
Aminodarone	↑/–	↑	↑	↑	↑	↑	↑
Sotalol	↑	↑			↑	↑	
Pirmenol		→	↑	↑		↑	↑
Cibenzoline		↑	↑	↑/–		↑/–	↑
Ethmozine							↑

Abbreviations : – = Minimal effect; SNRT = Sinus node recovery time; HP = His-Purkinje

RELATIVE EFFECTIVENESS AND SAFETY OF CALCIUM ANTAGONISTS IN CLINICAL CONDITIONS

	Nifedipine		Diltazem		Verapanil	
Coronary artery spasm (Prinzmetal's)	++++	S	++++	S	++++	S
Angina						
Stable	++	RS*	++	RS	+++	RS
Combined with beta-blocker	++++	S	+++	RS	++++	RS
With						
— chronic obstructive lung disease	++	RS	+	RS	++	RS
— heart failure	+	RS		CL		CI
— bradycardia	++	RS		CI		CI
— sick sinus	++	RS		CI		CI
— hypertension	+++	S	++	S	++	S
— hypertension plus beta-blocker	++++	S	+++	S	+++	RS
— unstable plus nitrates	+++	R/CI**	++	RS**	++	RS**
— unstable plus beta-blocker	+++	RS	++	RS	++	R/CI
— unstable threatened infarction	++	CI		R/CI		R/CI

RELATIVE EFFECTIVENESS AND SAFETY OF CALCIUM ANTAGONISTS IN CLINICAL CONDITIONS

	Nifedipine		Diltazem		Verapamil	
Aortic or mitral regurgatation	++	RS		CI		CI
Raynaud's phenomenon	+++	S	+	S	++	S
Severe aortic stenosis		CI		CI		CI
Obstructive cardiomyopathy		CI	+	RS	++	RS
Supraventricular tachycardia		O	++	RS	++++	RS
Atrial flutter-fibrillation		O	++	RS	++	RS

+++	=	most effective	S = safe
+	=	may be effective	RS = relatively safe in selected patients
O	=	not effective	R/CI = relative contraindication
CI	=	contraindicated	** = may increase infarction rate and mortality
*	=	rare increase in angina, carefully titrate dose	

PHARMACOKINETIC PROPERTIES OF DIFFERENT ACE INHIBITORS

Name	Prodrug	Hepatic metabolism binding (%)	Plasma t1/2 (hr.)	Plasma Protein (mg)	Excretion	Usual dose
1. *SH-containing*						
Captopril	No	+	< 2	30	Renal	25 TID (CHF) 25 BID (HT)
2. *Non SH-containing*						
Benazepril	Yes	+	> 20	> 90	Renal	upto 80 OD(HT)
Cilazepril	Yes	+	8-24	Not known	Renal	2-5 OD (HT) 5 OD (CHF)
Enalapril	Yes	+	> 30	< 50	Renal (75%)	10 BID (HT) 5 BID (CHF)
Lisinopril	Yes	—	7-12	No	Renal	10-20 OD (HT) 5-20 OD (CHF)

PHARMACOKINETIC PROPERTIES OF DIFFERENT ACE INHIBITORS (Contd...)

Name	Prodrug (hr.)	Hepatic metabolism binding (%)	Plasma 1/2	Plasma Protein (mg)	Excretion	Usual dose
Perindopril	Yes	+	> 30	20	Renal	2-4 OD (HT, CHF)
Quinapril	Yes	+	2	97	Renal	10-40 OD (HT) 5-20 OD (CHF)
Ramipril	Yes	+	> 30	56	Renal	2.5-10 OD (HT) 2.5 OD (CHF)
3. *Phosphoryl contuining*						
Fosinopril	Yes	+	12	90	Renal & Hepatic	10-40 OD (HT)

WHICH DRUG TO CHOOSE AS INITIAL OR MONO-THERAPY FOR MILD HYPERTENSION

Patient Type	Beta-Blocker	Diuretic	ACE-I	C	CA	Alpha-Blocker	Alpha Beta-Blocker
Age <65							
relatively healthy	1	2	2	3	3	4	3
Blacks	2	1	3	3	3	3	2
Any age group :							
Ischemic heart	1	3	3	4	2	RCI	3
LVH	1	3	2	3	3	RCI	3
Aneurysms	1	3	2	3	3	RCI	2
Cerebral ischemia	1	2	2	3	2	4	3
Heart failure	CI	1	1	RCI	3	4	CI
Diabetes :							
Insulin-dependent	RCI	3	1	2	3	2	3
Prone to hypoglycemia	CI	3	1	2	3	2	3
Gout	1	RCI	2	2	2	2	3
Hyperlipdemia :							
Mild	1	2	1	2	2	2	3
Moderate	2	3	1	2	2	2	2
Smokers: won't quit	1*	2	2	3	3	4	3
Osteoporosis		1**	2	3	4	4	3

WHICH DRUG TO CHOOSE AS INITIAL OR MONO-THERAPY FOR MILD HYPERTENSION

Patient Type	Beta-Blocker	Diuretic	ACE-I	C	CA	Alpha-Blocker	Alpha Beta-Blocker
Women age > 45	1	1	2	3	3	4	3
Chronic lung	CI	1	2	2	3	CI	
***	2+	1+	4+	2+	4+	2+	3+
↑	Yes	Yes	Yes	No	No	No	No

ACE-I = Angiotensin-converting enzyme inhibitor

CA = Calcium antagonist

C = Contraindicated

CI = Contraindicated

RCI = Relative contraindication

LVH = Left ventricular hypertrophy

* = Use a non-hepatic metabolized beta-blocker

** = Increases bone mineral density

*** = Cost 4+ = expensive, 1 + = low cost

-= proven effective, given alone, once daily

± = enalapril

1 = first choice; 4 = poor choice

HEMODYNAMIC AND ELECTROPHYSIOLOGIC EFFECTS OF CALCIUM ANTAGONISTS

	Nifedipine	*Diltiazem*	*Verapamil*
Coronary dilatation	++	++	++
Peripheral dilatation	+++	+	++
Negative inotropic	+	+	+++
AV conduction	++	+++	++++
Heart rate	⇑	↓++	↓↔
Blood pressure	++++	++	++
Sinus node depression	↩→	+	++
Cardiac output	++	↩→	↩→

+	=	inimal effect	++++	=	maximal effect
++	=	no significant change	↓	=	decrease
↑	=	increase			

COMPARISON BETWEEN HEPARIN AND DICOUMAROL

	Heparin	*Dicoumarol*
Source	Natural (mast cell)	Synthetic
Actions anticoagulant	Physiological	Not physiological
	Antithrombin	Antiprothrombin
	Antithromboplastin	Antifactor VII, IX, X
	Acts to vitro and vivo	Acts in vivo
Onset	Immediate	Delayed
Duration	3 hours	3 to 7 days
Coagulation time	+++	+
Prothrombin time	+	+++
Dose control	Coagulation time	Prothrombin time
Administration	IV	Oral
Antidote	Protamine sulph IV Hexadimethrine	Fresh blood Vitamin K I.V.
Use	Coronary thrombosis Surgery on C.V.S. Operation of artificial kidney	Coronary thrombosis Pulmonary embolism Post operative thrombophlebitis

PROPERTIES OF IMPORTANT CARDIOVASCULAR DRUGS USED IN SHOCK

	Dopamine	Isoprenaline	Noradrenaline
Action	Low dose rates stimulate beta and high dose rates stimulate alpha receptors. Direct action dilates coronary, splanchnic and renal arteries	Stimulates beta receptors	Stimulates mainly alpha receptors
Cardiac output	Increased With With low high	↑	May increase
Peripheral resistance	dose dose → ↑	↓	↑
Urine output	Increases ++	Increases +	May increase
Infusion rate	2-20 µg/kg/min (low) 2025 µg/kg/min (high)	Less than 10 µg/min	1-5 µg/min
Comments	Drug of choice after myocardial infarction. May be used in other types of shock.	Useful in later stages of bacteremic shock. Cardiac action not inhibited by acidosis. Never use in shock after myocardial infarction.	General purpose vasopressor. Never use in shock after myocardial infarction. Action inhibited by acidosis

DRUGS USED AT CARDIAC ARREST

Drug	Dose	Action
Adrenaline 1 : 1000 (1mg/ml) 1 : 1000 (1mg/10 ml)	100 μg-1 mg i.v. or intracardiace	α and β-receptor stimulator. May cause ventricular tachycardia or fibrillation
Atropine 0.5-1.2 mg/ml	0.6-1.8 mg	Mainly via vagal nucleus, 'blocks vagus'. Decreases vagal tone and increases heart rate especially when due to sinus bradycardia.
Bretylium	5-10 mg/kg	Prolongs action potential. 'pharmacological defibrillator'. used in refractory ventricular fibrillation.
Calcium chloride 10% (0.68 mmol Ca++/ml)	10 ml	Inotropic. May cause ventricular asystole in tonic contraction
Calcium gluconate 10% (0.225 mmol Ca++/ml)		
(Physical incompatibility with bicarbonate)		
Diphenylhydantoin (phenytoin) 50 mg/ml	50-100 mg	Membrane stabilisation. Especially in digitalis induced arrhythmia. Disopyramide or mexiletine may be preferred.
Disopyramide 10 mg/ml	50-150 mg	Membrane stabilisation. ↓ tendency for tachyarrhythmias (inc. digitalis-induced)

DRUGS USED AT CARDIAC ARREST (Contd...)

Drug	Dose	Action
Lignocaine 2% 20 mg/ml	100 mg	Membrane stabilisation ↓ tendency for tachyarrhythmias
Mexiletine 25 mg/ml	100 mg induced)	Membrane stabilisation. ↓ tendency for tachyarrhythmias (inc. digitalis-
Practolol 5 mg 2 mg/ml	5 mg	β-blocker - for SVT Do not give VERAPAMIL subsequently
Sodium bicarbonate 8.4% 1 mmol/ml (incompatible with Ca++)	50 mmol	Corrects acidosis Allows easier recovery of spontaneous activity
Verapamil 2.5 mg/ml NOT with b-blockers	5-10 mg	Calcium antagonist. Supraventricular tachyarrhythmias such as Wolff-Parkinson-White syndrome

THE VASODILATORS USED IN THE TREATMENT OF HYPERTENSION CAN BE CLASSIFIED BASED ON THEIR SITE AND MECHANISM OF ACTION AS FOLLOWS

1. *Drugs acting on the C.N.S.*

    (a) Clonidine, (b) Alpha methyldopa, (c) Mebutamate.

2. *Ganglion blocking drugs*

    (a) Quaternary ammonium compounds e.g. Hexamethonium, Pentolinium.

    (b) Monosulfonium compounds e.g. Trimethaphan

    (c) Secondary and tertiary amine e.g. Mecamylamine and Pempidine.

3. *Drugs preventing the release of catecholamines*

    (a) Bretylium, (b) Guanethidine, (c) Bethanidine, (d) Debrisoquine.

4. *Catecholamine depletors.*

    (a) Bretylium, (b) Rescinnamine, (c) Deserpidine.

5. *Drugs acting directly on the blood vessels.*

    (a) Prazosin, (b) Diazoxide, (c) Hydralazine, (d) Sodium nitroprusside, (e) Minoxidil

6. *Drugs acting by reducing the plasma volume.*

    (a) Thiazide diuretics, (b) Fursemide, (c) Spironolactones

7. *Drugs acting on the afferent nerve endings*

    Veratrum alkaloids

8. *Drugs blocking renin-angiotensin aldosterone axis.*

    (a) Blocking renin release eg Beta blockers

    (b) Blocking conversion of angiotensin I to angiotensin II (blocking enzyme ACE) eg. Captopril, Enalapril, Lisinopril.

    (c) Competitive blocking angiotensin II at vascular receptor sites eg saralasin

    (d) Counteracting aldosterone eg. spironolactone

9. *Miscellaneous.*

    MAO inhibitor (Pargyline), calcium channel blockers (Diltiazem, Nifedipine)

STREPTOKINASE THERAPY

Indications

Acute Myocardial infarction

* onset of symptoms within 24 hours
* clinically definite infarct

Major pulmonary embolism

* Persisting hypotension despite treatment with oxygen, heparin and i.v. colloid
* Confined by pulmonary angiography

Problems

* Allergic reaction (fever or urticaria) (give chlorpheniramine 10 mg i.v. and hydrocortisone 100 mg i.v.)
* Oozing from puncture sites (use a 22 gauge needle and compress the site for 10 min. and i.v. lines should be inserted via antecubital fossa)
* Uncontrolled bleeding (stop infusion, transfuse whole fresh blood or fresh frozen plasma and give Tranexamic acid 100 mg/kg i.v. over 10 min)

CONTRAINDICATIONS TO STREPTOKINASE THERAPY

1. Previous treatment with streptokinase (more than 5 days and upto 6 months) (altephase [plasminogen activator] can be used instead)
2. Active bleeding
3. Stroke within 2 months
4. Recent (within 10 days)
   * Major surgery
   * Chilbirth
   * Invasinve procedure (eg liver biopsy)
   * Trauma (including cardiopulm. resuscitation)
   * GI haemorrhage
5. Intravascular thrombus (in ventricular or aortic aneurysm)
6. Pregnancy (menstration is not a contraindication)
7. Haemostatic defect
8. Diabetic proliferative retinopathy
9. Severe hypertension (systolic more than 200 mm Hg, diastolic more than 110)
10. Bacterial endocarditis.

TREATMENT REGIMEN OF STREPTOKINASE

1.	Acute MI	*	Add 1.5 million units to 100 ml dextrose 5% or normal saline and infuse over 60 min.
		*	Give aspirin 150 mg p.o
2.	Major pulmonary	*	Add 2.5 lac units to 100 ml of dextrose 5% or normal saline and infuse over 30 min. Then give 1 lac
	embolism		units/hr for 24 hrs.
		*	It is convenient but not essential to infuse via the angiography catheter (which should be left in place because of risk of bleeding from puncture site)
		*	Check the thrombin time (TT) or kaolin-cephalin clotting time (KCCT) 3-4 hours after stopping streptokinase when TT/KCCT are less than twice control start a heparin infusion.

GENERATIONS OF THROMBOLYTIC AGENTS

First Generation :

> Streptokinase

> Urokinase

Second generation

> Recombinant tissue plasminogen activator (rt-PA)

> Anistreplase (APSAC)

> Prourokinase (Scu - PA)

Third generation

> Synergistic combination (eg tPA + Scu PA)

> Hybrids

> Fibrin antibody conjugated Scu - PA, tPA

CLASSIFICATION OF COAGULANTS

1. **Local haemostatics** (Styptics) : Control bleeding when applied locally.

   (a) Physical agents : Oxidised cellulose, gelatin sponge.

   (b) Vasoconstrictors : Adrenaline (applied locally).

   (c) Astringents (precipitation of proteins at site of bleeding). Vegetable astringent (contains tannic acid). Metallic astringent (Ferric chloride solution, alum).

   (d) Snake venom, trypsin (promotes formation of thrombin from prothrombin). Russel viper venom (stimulates thrombokinase).

   (e) Thrombin, fibrin foam (sponge of human fibrin saturated with thrombin solution; used in brain and lung surgery).

   (f) Oxidised cellulose : Formation of clot by cellulosic acid.

   (g) E-amino caproic acid : inhibitor of plasminogen activation and plasmin.

2. **Coagulants used systemically.**

   (a) Vitamin K : Increases formation of prothrombin, factor VII, IX, X

   (b) Blood transfusion, serum, plasma.

   (c) Miscellaneous : Calcium, congored, Vitamin C, Carbazochrome.

CLASSIFICATION OF ANTICOAGULANTS.

1. Agents which prevent action of ionic calcium : Oxalate, Fluoride, Citrate (Act in vitro only).

2. Drugs which interfere with synthesis of prothrombin and factor VII in liver, (Effective in vivo only).

   (a) Coumarin compounds eg. Dicoumarol, Warfarin, Ethylbiscoumacetate, Cyclocoumarol.

   (b) Indandione compounds e.g. phenindione, diphenadione.

3. Drugs inhibiting conversion of prothrombin to thrombin and interfering action of thrombin on fibrinogen : Heparin, (acts in vivo and vitro).

INTERACTION OF ANTICOAGULANTS

Increased anticoagulant Effect

Tetracycline

Trichloroethanol

Clofibrate

Probenecid

Alcohol

Talbutamide

Thyroxine

Phenformin

Phenylbutazone

Diphenhydramine

Liquid paraffin

Aspirin (antirheumatics) (high doses)

Sulfonamide

Chloramphenicol

Phenytoin

Quindine

Anabolic steroids

Quinine

Chlorpromazine

Decreased Effect

Cholestyramine

Nitrazepam

Griseofulvin

Vit. K

Griseofulvin

Antirheumatics

Oral contraceptives

ENDOCRINOLOGY

RELATIVE POTENCIES OF ADRENAL STEROIDS
Approximate Relative Potency

	Compound (tablet strength)	Anti-inflammatory (Glucocorticoid) Effect	Sodium retaining (Mineralocorticoid) Effect	Equivalent Dosage (for Anti-inflammatory Effect)
Cortisone	25 mg	0.8	1	25 mg
Hydrocortisone	20 mg	1.0	1	20 mg
Prednisolone and prednisone	5mg	4	0.8	5mg
Methyl-Prednisolone	4 mg	5	minimal	4 mg
Triamicinolone	4 mg	5	none	4 mg
Dexamethasone	0.5 mg	30	minimal	0.75 mg
Betamethasone	0.5 mg	30	negligible	0.7 mg
Paramethasone	2 mg	10	negligible	2 mg
Deoxycortone	—	negligible	50	—
Fludrocortisone	0.1 mg	15	150	—
Aldosterone	—	none	500	—

GLUCOCORTICOID CORTICOSTEROIDS

	Equivalent dosage (mg)	Mean dose to suppress HPA (mg/day)	Half-life in plasma (h)	Half-life of pharmacological effect (h)
Hydrocortisone	20	15-30	1.5	8-12
Cortisone	25	20-35	1.5	8-12
Prednosolone	5	7.5-10	3+	18-36
Prednisone	5	7.5-10	3+	18-36
Methylprednisolone	4	7.5-10	3+	18-36
Dexamethasone	0.75	1-1.5	5+	36-54
Triamcinolone	4	7.5-10	3+	18-36
Betamethasone	0.6	1-1.5	5+	36-54

Progestins can also be classified on the basis of their biological characteristics :

I.   *Pure progestins* e.g. Progesterone, Dehydrogesterone, Esters of 17-alpha hydroxyprogesterone, Chlormadinone and Megestrol.

II. *True progestins with possible androgenic effects* e.g. Medroxyprogesterone, Norgestrel,

III. *Progestins with androgenic effects* e.g. Norethisterone.

IV. *Progestins with estrogenic effects* e.g. Norethynodrol.

V.   *Steroids of uncertain status* e.g. Ethynodiol diacetate.

ELECTROLYTE EXCRETION PATTERN FOLLOWING DIURETICS

Drug	Urinary electrolytes				Effect of	
	Na	K	Cl	HCO3	Acidosis	Alkalosis
Organic Mercurials	+++	*	+++	—	—	Decreased
Acetazolamide	++	++	—	++	Decreased	—
Thiazodes	+++	++	++	*	Decreased	—
Frusemide	+++	++	+++	+	—	—
Ethacrynic acid	+++	++	+++	—	—	—
Spironolactone	+	*	+	+	—	—
Triamterene	++	*	++	+	—	—
Aminophylline	++	—	++	—	Decreased	—
Mannitol	++	—	++	—	—	—

* denotes potassium retention   — denotes no change

EQUIVALENT DOSES OF CORTICOSTEROIDS

Drug	Dose
Cortisone	25 mg
Hydrocortisone	20 mg
Prednisone and prednisolone	5 mg
Methylyprednisolone	4 mg
Dexamethasone	0.75 mg
Betamethasone	0.70 mg

USES OF RADIOISOTOPES IN MEDICINE

Radioisotopes are now extensively used in various branches of medicine for diagnostic, research and therapeutic purposes. The common uses of isotopes are :

I.   Haematology :

(a)   Measurement of blood volume, red cell survival, gastrointestinal blood loss by using red cells labelled with Chromium-51.

(b)   Iron absorption, erythropoiesis and iron kinetics by using 59Fe (iron).

(c)   Vitamin B12 absorption studies with radiocobalt (57Co) labelled B12; folic acid absorption studies by using tritiated (319) folic acid.

II.   Chemical Pathology :

(a)   Studies on sodium, potassium, water and chloride metabolism using 24NaCl, 42 KCl, tritiated water and radio bromide.

(b)   Plasma protein metabolism using I^{131}, human serum albumin; amino acid metabolism with 14C or 35S labelled amino acids.

(c)   Fat absorption studies by using labelled I^{131} tiolein and oleic acid.

(d)   Calcium kinetics by using Calcium-47.

III. Cardiovascular System :

(a) I^{131} and I^{132} uptake studies

(b)   Localization of thyroid tissue by using the same isotopes

V.   Urinary System :

(a)   Kidney localization by Hg203 labelled chlormerodrin.

(b)   Renal clearance studies by using I^{131} Sodium iodohippurate.

VI.   Tissue Scanning :

I^{131} and 99m Tc for thyroid scanning; Indium-113 m for liver, lung, brain, kidney and bone marrow scanning; Technetium-99-m for liver, brain and spleen scanning; 75-Sclenomethionine for parathyroid and pancreas scanning and macro-aggregated RIHSA (MAA-I131) for lung scanning.

VII. In assay procedures :

For biologicals and drugs e.g radioimmunoassay.

VIII. For Therapy :

(a) I^{131} for thyrotoxicosis and thyroid carcinoma.

(b)   Radiogold (Au192 and Cobalt-60 for the treatment of certain malignancies and secondaries.

(c)   P32 in the treatment of polycythemia vera.

(d)   Yitrium-90 for radiation hypophysectomy.

(e)   Tantallum-182 for carcinoma of bladder.

CHEMOTHERAPY

CLASSIFICATION OF ANTIBIOTICS ACCORDING TO SPECTRA

1. **Antibiotics mainly effective against gram +ve bacteria**
   (a) Those employed for systemic infections

   e.g Penicillins, Erythromycin, Lincomycin, Oleandomycin, Vancomycin, Novobiocin & Fucidin.

   (b) Those employed topically e.g. Bacitracin.

2. **Antibiotics mainly effective against gram + ve bacteria**
   (a) Those employed for systemic infections

   e.g. Streptomycin, Kanamycin, Gentamicin, Colistin, Polymyxin B & Cycloserine.

   (b) Those used locally in the intestines e.g. Paromomycin

3. **Antibiotics effective against both gram +ve and gram -ve bacteria**
   (a) Those employed for systemic infections

   e.g. Ampicillin; Amoxycillin, Carbenecillin, Cephalosporins, Rifamycins

   (b) Those employed topically

   e.g. Neomycin, Tyrothricin and Framycetin

4. **Antibiotics effective against both gram +ve and gram +ve bacteria, rickettsiae and chlamydia**

   e.g. Tetracyclines and Chloramphenicol.

5. **Antibiotics effective against acid fast bacilli**

   e.g. Streptomycin, Cycloserine, Viomycin, Capreomycin, Kanamycin, Rifampicin.

6. **Antibiotics effective against protozoa**

   e.g. Paromomycin, Tetracyclines, Fumagillin

7. **Antibiotics effective against fungi**

   e.g. Nystatin, Amphotericin B, Griseofulvin, Hamycin and Pimaricin

CLASSIFICATION OF CEPHALOSPORINS

First Generation
Cephaloridine
Cephalothin
Cefazolin*
Cephradine
Cephalexin (oral)
Cefadroxil (oral)

Second Generation
Cefamandole
Cefotetan
Cefoxitin
Cefonicid
Cefuroxime
Axetil (oral)

Third Generation
Moxalactum
Cefotaxime
Ceftriaxone
Cefoperazone
Ceftazidine
Ceftizoxime
Cefsulodin

NEWER 4-QUINOLONES AND THEIR INDICATIONS

1.	Acrosoxacin (Rosoxacin)	—	Gonorrhoea
2.	Cinoxacin	—	UTI
3.	Enoxacin	—	UTI, skin infections, gonorrhoea
4.	Ciprofloxacin	—	Gram -ve and some gram +ve infections
5.	Norfloxacin	—	URI, gram - ve infections
6.	Ofloxacin	—	Like ciprofloxacin

MECHANISMS OF ACTIONS OF ANTIMICROBIAL AGENTS

Interference with cell wall synthesis :
Penicillins, Cephalosporins, Bacitracin and Cycloserine.

Damage to the cytoplasmic membrane :
Polymyxins, Colistin and Polyene antibiotics

Inhibition of protein synthesis and impairment of the function of ribosomes :
Aminoglycosides, Tetracyclines, Chloramphenicol, Macrolide antibiotics and Lincomycin.

Interfering with the transcription of genetic information on the ribosomes :
Rifamipicin

Antimetabolite action :
Sulfonamides, Sulfones, PAS, INH, Ethambutol and Trimethoprim.

DOSES OF ANTIMICROBIAL AGENTS IN RENAL FAILURE

Agent	Loading dose	Maintenance dose	Interval between doses		
				Oliguria	Azotemia
Gentamicin	2 mg/kg	1 mg/kg.		2-3 days	1 day
Kanamycin sulfate	15 mg/kg	7.5 mg/kg		3-4 days	2 days
Streptomycin	15 mg./kg	7.5 mg/kg		3-4 days	2 days
Colistimethate sodium	5 mg/kg	2. mg/kg		3-4 days	2 days
Polymyxin B sulfate	2.5 mg/kg	1.25 mg/kg		3-4 days	2 days
Tetracycline	0.5 gm	0.25 gm		3-4 days	2 days
Chloramphenicol	0.5 gm.	0.5 gm.		6 hours	6 hours
Ampicillin	0.5 gm.	0.25 gm.		12 hours	6 hours
Cephalothin sodium	1.0-2.0	0.5-1.0 gm		24 hours	12 hours

COMMONLY USED BACTERIOSTATIC AND BACTERICIDAL DRUGS

Bactericidal	Bacteriostatic
Penicillin	Sulfonamides
Streptomycin	Nitrofurans
Polymyxin, colistin	Erythromycin
Kanamycin	Tetracyclines
Neomycin	Chloramphenicol
Cephalosprins	Lincomycin
Bacitracin	Triacetyloleandomycin
Isoniazid	Novobiocin
Gentamicin	PAS

THE DRUGS USED IN CHEMOTHERAPY OF AMOEBIASIS MAY BE CLASSIFIED CLINICALLY AS FOLLOWS :

I. *Drugs used only in intestinal amoebiasis :* Emetine bismuth iodide, halogented oxyquinolines, pentavalent organic arsenicals, antibiotics, diloxanide furoate, chlorphenoxamide secnidazole.

II. *Drugs used in both intestinal and extraintestinal amoebiasis :* Emetine, dehydroemetine, metronidazole, phanquone.

III. *Drugs used only in extraintestinal amoebiasis :* Chloroquine.

An alternative chemical classification is :

I. *Emetine group e.g :* Emetine, dehydroemetine and its resinate, emetine bismuth iodide.

II. *Quioline derivatives :*

(a) Halogenated hydroxyquinolines : Diiodohydroxyquinolines, iodochlorohydroxyquinolines, chiniofon sodium, broxyquinoline, chlorohydroxyquinolones.

(b) 4-aminoquinolines : Chloroquine, amodiaquine.

III. *Organic arsenicals :* Carbarsone and glycobiarsol.

V. *Miscellaneous :* Diloxanide furoate, chlorphenoxamide, niridazole, metronidazole, phanquone, secnidazole, or nidazole

COMMON FORMS OF HELMINTHIASIS AND THE DRUGS USED IN THEIR TREATMENT

Infestation	Drug of choice	Other drugs used
Taeniasis	Mepacrine	Chloroquine, paromomycin,
	Niclosamide	Dichlorophen
D. latum	Niclosamide	Mepacrine, Paromomycin,
		Dichlorophen
H. nana	Paromomycin	Niclosamide, Mepacrine,
		Dichlorophen
Taeniasis	Mepacrine	Chloroquine, paromomycin,
	Niclosamide	Dichlorophen
D. latum	Niclosamide	Mepacrine, Paromomycin,
		Dichlorophen
H. nana	Paromomycin	Niclosamide, Mepacrine,
		Dichlorophen
Ascariasis	Piperazine	Pyrantel, Bephenium,
	Tetramisole	Mebendazole
Ancylostomiasis	Tetrachloroethylene	Mebendazole, Pyrantel,
	Bephenium	Tetramisole, Bitoscanate
Oxyuriasis	Viprinium	Mebendazole, Pyrantel, Piperazine
Trichuriasis	Mebendazole	Thiabendazole, Bephenium
Schistosomiasis	Lucanthone	Trivalent antimonals, Amphotalide,
		Niridazole
Filariasis	Diethylcarbamazine	Carbarsone
Dracontiasis	Metronidazole	Thiabendaole
	Niridazole	
Strongyloidiasis	Thiabendole	Mebendazole

ANTIBACTERIAL CHEMOTHERAPY OF CHOICE

PENICILLINS :

Penicillin G : is the chemotherapy of choice in :
* Pneumococci
* Streptococci
* Meningococci
* Non-Beta-lactomase-producing staphylococci
* Gonococci
* Treponema pallidum
  Bacillus anthracis
* Clostridia
* Actinomyces
* Listeria
* Bacteroides (except Bacteroides fragilis)
* Leptospira

Benzathine Penicillin :
* Beta-hemolytic streptococcal pharyngitis
* Prophylaxis of rheumatics (against group A streptococci)
* Early syphilis

Aminopenicillins : (Ampicillin or Amoxicillin)
* H. influenzae
* Enterococcus faecalis
* Diverticulitis
* Bacterial exacerbations of bronchitis
* Community-acquired pneumonia

Penicillinase-resistant penicillins :
(Methicillin, Nafcillin etc.)
* Beta-lactamase-producing staphylococci
* Coagulase-negative staphylococci
* S. pyogenes
* S. pneumoniae

Carboxy Penicillins : (Carbenicillin and Ticarcillin)
* P. aeruginosa
* Indole-positive proteus sps.
* Non-Beta-lactamase-producing haemophilus, N. meningitidis, and N. gonorrhoeae

Ureido Penicillins :

(Azlocillin, mezlocillin etc.)

* Pseudomonas infections

Amdinocillin :

* Gram-negative species

Cephalosporins :

I first-Generation :

Oral Compounds	Parenteral Agents
Cephalexin	Cephalothin
Cephradine	Cephrapirin
Cepfadroxil	Cefazolin
Cefaclor	Cephradine

* Inhibit group A, B, C, and G Streptococci
* Most viridans group streptococci

II Second-Generation :

Oral : Cefuroxime axetil

IV : Cefamandole

Cefuroxime

Cefonicid

Cefoxtin

III Third-Generation :

Aminothiazolyl iminomehoxy

Cephalosporins :

Cefotaxime

Ceftizoxime

Cefmenoxime

Ceftriaxone

* Cefoxitin—Bacteroides fragilis, abd. sepsis
* Cefrulodin—Ps. aeruginosa
* Ceftazidime—Gram negative bacilli

Vancomycin is the drug of choice in :

* Methicillin-resistant staphylococci
* Antibiotic-associated colitis caused by C. difficile
* E. faecalis endocarditis in penicillin - Allergic patients
* Prevention of bacterial endocarditis in patients allergic to penicillin with prosthetic heart valve

Aminoglycosides :
* Enterobacteriaceae E. coli, Klebsiella, serratia, enterobacter
* Gentamicin, tobramycin, amikacin, sisomicin and netilmicin inhibit P. aeruginosa except kanamycin
* Acinetobacter
* Proteus vulgaris and other sps.
* Serratia, Providencia

Streptomycin :
* Plague
* Tularemia
* Brucellosis
* Selective cases of TB
* Endocarditis cause by S. faecalis or Streptococcus viridans
* Granuloma inguinale

Gentamicin :
* Gram-negative infections

Neomycin : (Topical and Oral use)
* Preparation for elective Bowel surgery
* Hepatic coma- to reduce coliform bacteria

Spectinomycin :
* Gonorrhea due to Penicillinase-producing strains

Tetracyclines : (Doxycycline)
* Rickettsiae (typhus fevers)
* Coxiella burnettii (Q fevers)
* Mycoplasma pneumoniae
* Chlamydial infectious
* LGV
* Psittacosis
* Non-gonococcal urethritis
* Brucellosis
* Bartanellosis
* Whipple's disease
* Tropical sprue
* Cholera .
* Psittacosis (Ornithosis)

Chloramphenicol :

* Symptomatic salmonella infection
* H. influenzae meningitis, laryngotracheitis or pneumonia that does not respond to ampicillin.
* Meningococcal infection in patients hypertensive to penicillin.
* Anaerobic or mixed inf. in CNS (brain abscess)
* Severe rickettsial infections

Erythromycin :
* Streptococcal pharyngitis in Penicillin-allergic patient.
* Skin infections in pregnancy
* Syphilis in pregnancy
* Legionella pneumophilia (pneumonia)
* M. pneumoniae
* Some Ureaplasma infections
* Campylobacter
* Diphtheria carriers

Co-trimoxazole :
* Paratyphoid
* Pneumocystis carnii
* Shigellosis
* Listeria meningitis in patients allergic to penicillins
* Prophylaxis in neutropenic children and chronic granulomatous disease of childhood.
* Prophylaxis in recurrent bacteriuria in woman with recurrent UTI

Clindamycin :
* Anaerobic pulmonary disease in patients failed to respond to penicillin

Metronidazole :
* B. fragilis (99% control)
* Fusobacterium (100%)
* Pseudomembranous enterocolitis due to C. difficile
* Serious anaerobic infections

Rifampin :
* Short-term treatment of tuberculosis combined with INH
* Prophylaxis for meningococcal meningitis and H. influenzae type B meningitis
* L. pneumophilia infection failed to respond to erythromycin

Amantadine Rimantadine :
* Influenza A (prophylaxis)
* Influenza A (therapy)

Acyclovir :
* Genital Herpes simplex
* Primary infection
* Recurrent infections (therapy)
  Recurrent infections (suppression)
* Mucocutaneous Herpes simplex in immunocompromised patients (prevention of recurrences during periods of intense immunosuppression)
* Herpes zoster ophthalmicus

Ribavirin :
* Respiratory syncytial virus

Ganciclovir :
* Cytomegalovirus infections

Acyclovir or Vidarabine
* Herpes simplex encephalitis
* Neonatal Herpes simplex
* Mucocutaneous Herpes simplex in immunocompromised patients (treatment)
* Varicella in immuno-compromised patients
* Herpes zoster in immuno-compromised patients

Trifluorothymidine or Vidarabien : Topical)
* Herpes simplex keratitis

ANTIFUNGAL THERAPY OF CHOICE

Topical agents :

Imidazole and triazoles :

(Clotrimazole, econazole and miconazole)
* Cutaneous candidiasis
* Tinea versicolor
* Ringworm
* Vulvovaginal candidiasis

Clotrimazole :
* Oral or oesophageal candidiasis

Tolnaftate and undecylenic acid :

* Ringworm

Nystatin :
* Oral thrush
* Vulvovaginal candidiasis

Systemic antifungals : Ketoconazole :
* Blastomycosis
* Histoplasmosis
* Paracoccidioidomycosis
* Chronic mucocutaneous
* Candidiasis

Amphotericin B :
* Histoplasmosis
* Blastomycosis
* Paracoccidioidomycosis
* Candidiasis
* Cryptococcosis

Flucytosine (5-flurocytosine) :
* Cryptococcosis
* Candidiasis
* Chromomycosis

Potassium iodide :
* Sporotrichosis

PARASITIC DISEASES

Bithinol :
* Paragonimiasis

Diethylcarbamazine :
* Filarial infections

Dehydroemetine :
* Tissue amebiosis

Diloxanide furoate :
* Intestinal amebiasis

Iodoquinol :
* Intestinal amebiasis
* Dientamoeba infections

Niclosamide :
Intestinal tapeworms
* Taenia solium

* Diphyllobothrium

Nifurtimox :
* Acute Chaga's disease

Pentamidine :
* Pneumocystosis
* Leishmaniasis
* Trypanosomiasis

Pyrantel pamoate :
* Pinworm infection
* Hookworm infection
* Ascariasis

Suramin :
* African trypanosomiasis
* Onchocerciasis

Praziquantel :
* Schistosomaisis
* Paragonimiasis
* Clonorchis
* Taenia saginata
* H. nana

Mebendazole :
* Echinococcus
* Trichuris
* Capillariasis

Thiabendazole :
* Toxocara
* Larva migrans
* Strongyloidosis
* Trichinella spiralis

Tinidazole :
* Giardiasis

Metronidazole :
Trichomoniasis
* Invasive amebiasis

ACTIVITY OF SOME IMPORTANT ANTIMICROBIALS

Benzyl-Penicillin	Gram-positive (except many staphs) and Gram-negative cocci, Some Gram-positive bacilli (C. diphtheria, clostridia, B. anthracis)
	Spirochaetes
Ampicillin	Gram-positive cocci (except many staphs) and bacilli
	Gram-negative bacilli except Klebsiella and many anaerobes
Cephalosporins	Gram-positive cocci
	Gram-negative bacilli
Gentamicin	Gram-negative bacilli, staphylococci (Note : streptococci and all anaerobes are resistant)
Tetracyclines	Gram-positive and Gram-negative cocci and bacilli
	Rickettsiae
	Chlamydia, Mycoplasma
	Spirochaetes
	E. histolytica
Sulphonamides and Cotrimoxazole	Gram-positive and Gram-negative cocci
	Gram-negative bacilli

RECOMMENDED DOSAGE OF ANTITUBERCULOSIS DRUGS ADMINISTERED ORALLY EXCEPT WHERE INDICATED

Drug	Daily dosage adults	children	Intermittent dosage adults
Isoniazid	5-10 mg/kg usually 300 mg	10-20 mg/kg up to 300 mg	15 mg/kg 2-3/wk.
Rifampicin	10 mg/kg up to 600 mg	10-20 mg/kg up to 600 mg	600 mg 2-3 wk
Pyrazinamide	20-40 mg/kg up to 1500-2000 mg or 3000 mg for re-treatment.	30 mg/kg up to 2000 mg	60 mg/kg 2-3 wk
Ethambutol	15-25 mg/kg	10-15 mg/kg	50 mg/kg 2-3 wk
Ethionamide or prothionamide	10-15 mg/kg up to 1 g	10-15 mg/kg up to 750 mg	NI
Cycloserine	10 mg/kg up to 1 g	10-20 mg/kg up to 500 mg	NI
Aminosalicyclic acid	250 mg/kg up to at least 12 g	300 mg/kg	NI
Streptomycin, caproomycin, kanamycin	15 mg/kg IM up to 1 g	20 mg/kg IM	1 g IM 2-3 wk
Thiocetazone	150 mg	NI	NI
Ciprofloxacin	1000-1500 mg	NI	NI
Ofloxacin	600 mg	NI	NI
Clofazimine	100-200 mg	NI	NI

Abbreviations : IM = intramuscular administration; NI = not indicated.

MAJOR ADVERSE REACTIONS TO ANTITUBERCULOSIS DRUGS

Drug	Adverse reaction
Isoniazid	Hepatitis, peripheral neuropathy, skin rashes, neurological disturbances
Rifampicin	Nausea, vomiting, abdominal cramps, diarrhoea; headache, drowsiness; transient elevation of ALT, AST and bilirubin; skin rashes, flu-like syndrome, renal failure, thrombocytopenia, haemolytic anaemia
Pyrazinamide	Hepatitis; skin rashes; arthralgia, gout, hyperuricaemia
Ethambutol	Retrobulbar neuritis
Ethionamide	Gastrointestinal irritation; excessive salivation, metallic taste in the mouth, anorexia, nausea, vomiting, diarrhoea; hepatitis; skin rashes, stomatitis, photosensitivity; goitre, acne, gynaecomastia, impotence, peripheral neuropathy, arthralgia
Cycloserine	Dizziness, headache, tremor, insomnia, slurred speech, depression, anxiety, psychosis, suicide attempts
Aminosalicylic acid	Anorexia, nausea, vomiting, diarrhoea; hepatitis; high sodium load; skin rashes
Streptomycin,	Vestibular and auditory toxicity; transient giddiness; numbness around the mouth;
capreomycin. kanamycin	skin rashes
Thioacetazone	Skin rashes; nausea, vomiting, diarrhoea; hepatitis; bone marrow depression, thrombocytopenia, agranulocytosis; dizziness, ataxia, vertigo, tinnitus
Ciprofloxacin, ofloxacin	Nausea, vomiting, diarrhoea; insomnia; headache; skin rashes
Clofazimine	Brownish pigmentation of skin; bowel obstruction; splenic infarction, gastrointestinal bleeding.

COMPOUNDS WHICH INTERACT WITH RIFAMPICIN

Compounds	Effects
Anticoagulants (warfarin)	↓ Serum Concentration
Cardiac Glycosides (digitoxin)	↓ Serum Concentration
Oral antidiabetics (tolbutamide)	↓ Serum Concentration
Oral contraceptive	↓ Efficacy
Corticosteroids	↓ Serum Concentration
Narcotic Analgesics (methadone,diamorphine)	↓ Serum Concentration; Withdrawal Syndrome
Dapsone	↑ Clearance
Cyclosporine	↓ Serum Concentration
Quinidine	↓ Peak Serum Concentration
Cholephils (bilirubin, bromosulphthalein)	↑ Serum concentration initially

FEW MISCELLANEOUS CONDITIONS—DRUG OF CHOICE

*	Diphtheria carier state	—	Erythromycin.
*	Chromo blastomycosis (Massy foot)	—	5-flurocytosine.
*	Sporotrichosis	—	Potassium iodide.
*	Coccidiodomycosis	—	Amphotericin B.
*	Anaphylaxis reaction	—	Adrenaline.
*	Asthmatic status	—	Adrenaline
*	Anginal attack	—	GTN (glyceryl trinitrate).
*	Complete heart block	—	Isoprenaline.
*	Carcinoid lung	—	Doxorubicin.
*	Myotonia congenita	—	Phenytoin, Quinidine etc.
*	Kawasaki disease	—	High dose of aspirin
*	Tropical splenomegaly	—	Proguanil.
*	Malignant hyperthermia	—	Diethyl carbamazine.
*	Narcolepsy	—	Amphetamine.
*	Cataplexy	—	Tricyclic antidepressants.
*	Capilariasis	—	Mebendazole.

*	*Toxocara*	— Thiabendazole.
*	*Larva migrans*	— Thiabendazole.
*	*Gnatho stomiasis*	— Bithionol
*	*Meningococcal carrier state*	— Rifampicin.
*	*Compylobacter diarrhoea*	— Erythromycin.
*	*Cerebral cysticercosis*	— Praziquantel
*	*Status epilepticus*	— Diazepam
*	*Obsessive compulsive disorder*	— Clomipramine/Fluoxetine
*	*Alcohol deaddiction*	— Buspirone
*	*Oriental sore*	— Sodium antimony
*	*Non-specific vaginitis*	— Tetracycline
*	*Non-specific vaginitis*	— Metronidazole
*	*Pneumocystis carinii*	— Cotrimoxazole
*	*Mycobacterium marinum*	— Minocycline
*	*Acute Gout*	— Colchicine

DRUG INTERACTIONS OF THEOPHYLLINE

* **↓ Theophyllinel Plasma levels** **(By ↑ metabolism)**

* **↑ Theophylline Plasma levels** **(By ↓ metabolism)**

↓ Theophyllinel Plasma levels (By ↑ metabolism)	↑ Theophylline Plasma levels (By ↓ metabolism)
Smoking	Erythromycin
Phenytoin	Ciprofloxacin
Rifampicin	Cimetidine
Phenobarb	OCP
Charcoal broiled meal milk	Allopurinol
	* (decrease dose to 2/3)

* **Theophylline ↑ effects of**   ↓ es effects of

Theophylline ↑ effects of	↓ es effects of
Furosemide	Phenytoin
Sympathomimetics	Lithium
Digitalis	
Oral anticoagulants	

* **Aminophylline injection should not be mixed in same infusion bottle/ syringe with —**
  ascorbic acid, chlorpromazine, promethazine, morphine, pethidine, pethidine, phenytoin, phenobarb, insulin, penicillin G, tetracyclines, erythromycin

THE DRUGS COMMONLY EMPLOYED IN THE TREATMENT OF MALIGNANT DISEASES CAN BE CLASSIFIED ACCORDING TO THEIR MODE OF ACTION AS FOLLOWS

I. *Alkylating agents :*

(a) Nitrogen mustards e.g. Mechlorethamine, Cyclophosphamide, Melphalan, Uracil mustard and Chlorambucil

(b) Ethylenimines e.g. Triethylenemelamine (TEM), Triethylene thiophosphoramide (Thio-TEPA).

(c) Alkyl Sulfonates e.g. Busulfan.

II. *Antimetabolites :*

(a) Folic acid antagonists e.g. Methotrexate (amethopterin).

(b) Purine antagonists e.g. 6-mercaptopurine, Azathioprine.

(c) Pyrimidine antagonists e.g. Fluorouracil, Fluorodeoxyuridine, Cytosine arabinoside.

III. *Radioactive isotopes* e.g. Radioiodine, Radiogold, Radiophosphorus.

IV. *Antibiotics* e.g. Actinomycin-D, Mitomycin-C, Rubidomycin, Adriamycin, Bleomycin, and Mithramycin.

V. *Miscellaneous agents :*

(a) Vinca alkaloids — Vinblastine, Vincristine.

(b) Others : Procarbazine, c,p DDD, 1-Asparaginase, Streptozotocin.

VI. *Hormones :* Androgens, estrogens, progestins and corticosteroids.

The following examples are included to give a general idea of the scope and range of cancer chemotherapy.

ENVIRONEMENTAL HAZARDS

* **Asbestos :**
    * Pulmonary effects
    * Mesotheliomas
* **Chloroform :**
    * Liver cancer
* **Chloromethyl Methyl Ether :**
    * Lung cancer
* **4,4' - Diaminodiphenyl Methane :**
    * Toxic hepatitis
* **Formaldehyde :**
    * Respiratory damage
    * Cancer
* **n-Hexane :**
    * Neuropathy
* **Kepone :**
    * Neurologic effects
* **Mirex :**
    * Liver cancer
* **Polybrominated Biphenyl (PBB) :**
    * Birth defects
* Liver cancer
* **Polychlorinated Biphenyl (PCB) :**
    * Birth defects
    * Liver cancer
    * Melanoma
* **Tetrachlorodibenzodoxin (TCDD) :**
    * Birth defects
* **Vinyl Chloride :**
    * Angiosarcoma of liver

SUBSTANCES ADSORBED BY CHARCOAL

Aconite	Imipramine	Opiates
Alcohol	Iodides	Oxalates
Antimony	Ipeca cuanha	Paracetamil
Arsenic	Isoniazid	Paraffin
Atropine	Lead	Parathione
Barbiturates	Malathion	Phenol
Camphor	Mefenamic acid	Phosphorus
Cantharides	Mercury	Potassium
Chloroquine	Methylene Blue	Permanganate
Chlorpheniramine	Morphine	Quinine
Chlorpromazine	Muscarine	Reserpine
Cocaine	Nicotine	Salicylate
Digitalis	Nortriptyline	Silver salts

TREATMENT OF AIDS-RELATD OPPORTUNISTIC INFECTIONS AND MALIGNANCIES

Infection	Treatment	Complication
P. carinii infection	Trimethoprim-sulfamethoxazole, 15 mg/kg/d (based on TMP component) orally or IV	Nausea, neutropenia, anemia, hepatitis drug rash, Stevens-Johnson syndrome
	Pentamidine, 3–4 mg/kg/d IV for 14-21 days pancreatitis, hepatitis.	Hypotension, hypoglycemia, anemia, neutropenia,
	Trimethoprim, 15 mg/kg/d orally, with dapsone, 100 mg/d orally, for 14-21 days	Nausea, rash, hemolytic anemia in G6PD-deficient patients.
		Methemoglobinemia (weekly levels should be <10% of total hemoglobin)
	Primaquine, 15-30 mg/d orally, and clindamycin, 300-900 mg every 6 hours orally, for 14-21 days (not well established)	Hemolytic anemia in G6PD-deficient patients. Methemoglobinemia, neutropenia, colitis.
	566C80 750 mg orally 3 times daily	Rash, elevated transminases, anemia neutropenia.
	Trimetrexate, 45 mg/m2 IV for 21 days (given with folinic acid)	Leucopenia, rash, mucositis
M. avium complex infection	Combination drug regimens in use: Clofazimine, 100 mg orally daily, plus—	Abdominal pain, discoloration of skin
	Ethambutol, 15 mg/kg/d orally (maximum, 1 g), plus—Rifampin, 10 mg/kg/d orally (maximu, 600 mg daily) plus—	Hepatitis, optic neuritis Rash, hepatitis
	Ciprofloxacin, 750 mg orally twice daily	Anaphylaxis, nausea, rash
	Amikacin, 7.5 mg/kg every 12-24 hours IV for 2-4 weeks (consider in addition to above treatments)	Nephrotoxicity, ototoxicity
	Clarithromycin, 750-1000 mg orally twice daily (also consider in addition to above drugs)3	Hepatitis

TREATMENT OF AIDS-RELATD OPPORTUNISTIC INFECTIONS AND MALIGNANCIES (Contd..)

Infection	Treatment	Complication
Toxoplasmosis	Pyrimethamine 100-200 mg orally as loading dose, followed by 50-75 mg/d, combined with sulfadiazine, 4-6 g orally daily in 4 divided doses, and folinic acid, 10 mg daily for 4-8 weeks; then pyrimethamine, 25-50 mg/d, with sulfadiazine, 2 g/d, and folinic acid, 5 mg/d	Leucopenia, rash
	Pyrimethamine, 100-200 mg orally as loading dose, foll-owed by 50-75 mg/d, combined with clindamycin, 600 mg orally every 6 hours for 4-8 weeks, and folinic acid, 10 mg orally daily then pyrimethamine, 25-50 mg/d, withclindamycin 300-600 mg. every 6 hours and folinic acid, 5 mg/daily	Abdominal pain, nausea, rash
Lymphoma	Combination chemotherapy (eg. modified CHOP, M-BACOD,4 with or without G-CSF or GM-CSF_5 Central nervous system disease; radiation treatment with dexamethasone for edema.	Nausea, vomiting, anemia, leucopenia, cardiotoxicity (with doxorubicin)
Cryptococcal meningitis	Amphotericin B, 0.6 mg/kg/d IV, to total dose of about 1.5 g. Maintenance therapy is with amphotericin B, 1 mg/kg/wk	For amphotericin B, fever, anemia, and azotemia
	Fluconazole, 400 mg orally as loading dose, then 200 mg orally daily	Hepatitis

TREATMENT OF AIDS-RELATD OPPORTUNISTIC INFECTIONS AND MALIGNANCIES (Contd...)

Infection	Treatment	Complication
Cytomegalovirus infection	Ganciclovir, 10mg/kg/d IV in 2 divided doses for 10 days, followed by 6 mg/kg 5 days a week indefinitely. (Decrease dose for renal impairment)	Neutropenia
	Foscarnet, 60 mg/kg IV 3 times daily (induction), followed by 90 mg/kg once daily. (Adjust for changes in renal function.)	Nausea, 1K, 1Ca, PO4
Esophageal candidiasis terfenadine	Ketoconazole, 200 mg orally twice daily for 2-4 weeks	Hepatitis, adrenal insufficiency: ventricular tachicardia when given with
	Ketoconazole, 100-200 mg daily for 2-4 weeks	Hepatitis
Herpes simplex infection	Acyclovir, 200 mg 5 times daily for 7-10 days; or acyclovir, 5 mg/kg IV every 8 hours for severe cases	Resistant herpes simplex with chronic therapy
	Foscarnet, 40 mg/kg IV every 4 hours, for acyclovir cases (Adjust for changes in renal function)	See above
Herpes zoster	Acyclovir, 800 mg orally 4-5 times daily for 7-10 days. Intervenous therapy at 15/mg/kg for ocular involvement, disseminated disease.	
	Foscarnet, 40 mg/kg IV every 8 hours for a acyclovir-resistant cases. (Adjust for changes in renal function)	See above
Kaposi's sarcoma Limited cutaneous disease	Observation, intralesional vinblastine	Inflammation, pain at site of injection

TREATMENT OF AIDS-RELATD OPPORTUNISTIC INFECTIONS AND MALIGNANCIES (Contd..)

Infection	Treatment	Complication
Extensive or aggressive cutaneous disease	Systemic chemotherapy (e.g alternating weekly vinca alkaloids) Alpha interferon (for patients with CD4 > 400 cells/ml and no constitutional symptoms) Radiation (amelioration or edema)	Bone marrow suppression, peripheral neuritis, flu-like syndrome
Visceral disease (e.g. pulmonary)	Combination chemotherapy	Bone marrow suppression

For moderate to severe P carinii infection (oxygen saturation < 90%) corticosteroids should be given with specific treatment.
CHOP= cyclophosphamide, doxorubicin, vincristine, and prednisone, Modified M-BACOD=methotrexate, bleomycin, doxorubicin, cyclophosphamide, vincristine, and dexamethasone.
CSF = granulocyte colony stimulating factor; GM-CSF = granulocyte macrophage colony stimulating factor

RESPONSE TO CHEMOTHERAPY

Group A   Tumours in which *striking response and significant benefit are common and life expectancy may become normal*

Childhood acute leukaemia (cure)
Choriocarcinoma (cure)
Wilm's sarcoma
Ewing's sarcoma
Seminoma
Prostatic carcinoma
(endocrine responsive)
Small cell bronchial carcinoma
Burkitt's tumour (cure)

Chronic granulocytic leukaemia
Chronic lymphocytic leukaemia
Hodgkin's disease (cure)
Follicular lymphoma
Reticulum cell sarcoma
Lymphosarcoma

Group B   Tumours in which *chemotherapy is less effective.*

Acute leukaemia in adults
Multiple myeloma
Cholangiocarcinoma

Breast carcinoma
Ovarian carcinoma

Group C   Tumours in which chemotherapy is *often ineffective,* or effective only when special techniques of administration are employed.

Cervix uteri carcinoma
Corpus uteri carcinoma
Melanoma
Gastrointestinal carcinoma
Hepatoma

Cerebral gliomata
Oropharyngeal carcinomas
Carcinoma of paranasal sinuses
Renal carcinoma

(Modified from WHO Technical Reports Nos 232 and 605)

CHOICE OF DRUGS IN MALIGNANCIES

Disease	Ist choice drugs	Alternatives and 2nd choice drugs
Acute leukaemias	Prednisolone Mercaptopurine	Asparaginase
Cyclophosphamide		
	Vincristine Methotrexate Daunorubicin (Rubidomycin) Doxorubicin (Adriamycin) Cytarabine	
Chronic granulocytic leukaemia	Busulphan	Mercaptopurine Hydroxyurea Melphalan
Chronic lymphocytic leukaemia	Chlorambucil Cyclophosphamide Prednisolone	
Hodgkin's lymphoma agents	Cyclophosphamide	Other alkylating
	Vinblastine Procarbazine Prednisolone	Vincrisline Bleomycin Dacarbazine, Doxorubicin
Burkitt's lymphoma	Cyclophosphamide	Carmustine Methotrexate
Other lymphomas	Prednisolone Cyclophosphamide Vincristine Bleomycin Doxorubicin Cytarabine Methotrexate	
Multiple myeloma	Melphalan Cyclophosphamide Prednisolone	Carmustine Doxorubicin Vincristine

CHOICE OF DRUGS IN MALIGNANCIES (Contd...)

Disease	1st choice drugs	Alternatives and 2nd choice drugs
Breast cancer	Hormones or anti-Hormones depending On endocrine status; Cyclophosphamide Methotrexate Fluorouracil Prednisolone	Doxorubicin Vincristine
Prostate cancer	Oestrogen	Alkylating agents
Ovary cancer	Melphalan Doxorubicin Cyclophosphamide	Cisplatin Chlorambucil Fluorouracil Methotrexate Doxorubicin
Endometrium cancer	A progestogen	
Cervix cancer	Mitomycin Methotrexate Cyclophosphamide	Bleomycin
Choriocarcinoma	Methotrexate	Actinomycin D Vinblastine Chlorambucil
Small cell carcinoma of bronchus	Doxorubicin Cyclophosphamide Vincristine Methotrexate Lomustine	Procarbazine Etoposide
Gastrointestinal cancers	Fluorouracil Mitomycin	Doxorubicin
Bladder cancer	Doxorubicin Cisplatin Thiotepa	Mitomycin Fluorouracil
Brain cancer	Carmustine Lomustine	Procarbazine Vincristine
Wilm's tumour	Actinomycin D Vincristine	Doxorubicin
Ewing's sarcoma	Cyclophosphamide Doxorubicin Vincristine Actinomycin D	
Osteogenic sarcoma	Doxorubicin Methotrexate with "Folinic acid rescue"	Cisplatin Melphalan

SOME ANTIVIRAL AGENTS IN DEVELOPMENT

Virus	Agents	Mechanism of action
HIV—1	Lamividine FTC	Nucleoside RT inhibitors
	Adefovir (PMEA)	"
	Nevirapine, delaviridine, loviride	Non-nucleoside RT inhibitors
	Saquinavir, indinavir	Protease inhibitors
Hepatitis B virus	Lamivudine, famciclovir, fialuridine	Nucleoside DNAP inhibitors
Herpes viruses	Colofovir (HPMPC)	"
	Lobucavir	"
Papilloma virus	Afovirsen	Antisene oligo-nucleolide
Rhinovirin	sICAM-1	Receptor decoy
	Pirodavir	Capsid-binding agents
Influenza virus	GG-167	Neuroaminidase inhibitor

CHARACTERISTICS OF TRUE AND PSEUDO CHOLINESTERASES

Property	Pseudo cholinesterase	True cholinesterase
Distribution	Plasma, liver & glial cells.	Neural structures, red blood cells and placenta.
Substrate	Hydrolyses benzoyl choline and does not hydrolyse Also succinylcholine.	Hydrolyses methacholine but does not hydrolyse benzoyl choline.
Physilogical role	Not known	It is concerned with destruction of acetylcho-line released at the nerve endings.

DIFFERENCES BETWEEN NEOSTIGMINE & PHYSOSTIGMINE

	Property	Physostigmine	Neostigmine
1.	Source	Physostigma venenosum	Synthetic
2.	Stability	Less stable	More stable
3.	Chemistry	Tertiary amine	Quaternary ammonium commpound
4.	Absorption from the G.I.T.	Good	Incomplete, oral dose 30 times higher than the subcutaneous dose
5.	Blood brain barrier	Crosses	Does not cross
6.	Skeletal muscle stimulatory action	No direct action	It has also got direct

DIFFERENCES BETWEEN NEOSTIGMINE & PHYSOSTIGMINE (Contd....)

	Property	Physostigmine	Neostigmine
7.	Toxicity of muscarinic actions on intestines	More than neostigmine	Less than physostigmine
9.	Therapeutic uses	(a) Used in atropine poisoning because crosses the blood brain barrier	(a) Not useful in atropine poisoning
		(b) Used topically in the eye because of better penetration	(b) Not preferred for ophthalmic use
		(c) Due to toxicity is not used systemically except	(c) Preferred for disorders of bladder, G.I.T. and skeletal muscles due to for atropine poisoning lesser toxicity.

SAFETY OF DRUGS IN PREGNANCY

Class of medication	Relatively sale to use in pregnancy	Limited data or fetal risk appear minimal	Evidence of fetal risk	Significant fetal risk avoid in pregnancy
Analgesics	Acetaminophen	Celexoxib Diclofenac Fentanyl Hydrocodone Hydromorphone Ibuprofen Ketoprofen Meperidine Morphine Naproxen Oxycodone Piroxican Rofecoxib Sulindac	Aspirin Codeine Etodolac Indomethacin Ketorolac Nabumetone Oxaprozin Propoxyphene Tramadol	
Articonvulsants	Magnesium Sulphate		Carbamazepine Clonazepam Ethosuximide Gabapentin Lamotrigine Tagabine Topiramate	Fosphenytoin Phenobarbital Phenytoin Primidone Valproic acid

SAFETY OF DRUGS IN PREGNANCY (Contd...)

Class of medication	Relatively safe to use in pregnancy	Limited data or fetal risk appear minimal	Evidence of fetal risk	Significant fetal risk avoid in pregnancy
Antidepresants/ Antipsychotics Antipsy Cotis		Bupropion Citalopram Fluoxetine Paroxetine Sertraline	Amitriptyline Desipramine Doxepin Haloperidol Imipramine Mirtazapine Nefazodone Nortriptyline Olanzapine Quetiapine Risperidone Thioridazine Trazodone Venlafaxine	Lithium Monoamine Oxidase Inhibitors
Antidiabetic Agents	Insulin	Acarbose Metformin Migitol	Glimepiride Glipizide Glyburide Pioglitazone Repaglinde Troglitazone	
Antiemetic	Doxylamine Meclizine Metoclopramide Pyridoxine	Chlorpromazine Dimenhydrinate Dolasetron Granisetron Ondansetron Prochlorperazine Promethazine Scopolamine Trimethobenzamide		
Antihistamines	Chlorphen- iramine Triprolidine	Astemizole Brompheniramine Cetrizine Clemastine Diphenhydramine Hydroxyzine Loratadine		
		Cholestyramine Colestipol	Fenofibrate Gemfibrate	HMG-Coa raductase inhibitors

SAFETY OF DRUGS IN PREGNANCY (Contd...)

Class of medication	Relatively sale to use in pregnancy	Limited data or fetal risk appear minimal	Evidence of fetal risk	Significant fetal risk avoid in pregnancy
Antimicrobials	Amoxycillin	Acyclovir Amoxicillin/	Amikacin Azithromycin	Fluroqinolones Ethmbutol
Strep-tomycin				
	Clavulanic acid	Aztreonam Chloramphenicol	Fluconazole Gentamicin	Tetracyclines
	Amphotericin-B Ampicillin Ampicillin/ Sulbactam Cephalosporins Clotrimazole (topical) Erythromycin Mezlocillin Miconazole (topical) Nitrofuratoin Nystain Oxacillin Penicillin Piperacillin Tazobactam Ticarcillliin\clavulanic acid	Clarithomycin Clindamycin Famciclovir Imipenemicil- astation Metronidazole Valacyclovir Vancomycin	Isoniazid Itraconazole Miconazole (Systemic) Pentamidine Pyrazinamide Rifampin Tobramycin Trimethoprim-sulfamethoxazole	
Antithrombotics		Clopidogrel Dalteparin Danapariod Dipyridamole Enoxaparin Heparin Lepirudin Ticlopidine	Aspirin	Warfarin
Cardiovascular drugs		Atenolol Clonidine Digoxin Doxazosin Hydralazine Labetalol Lidocaine Methyldopa Metoprolol	Amlodipine Diltiazem Felodipine Nicardipine Nifedipine Nitrates Verapamil	Angiotensin Converting Enzyme Inhibitors Angiotension II-receptor Antagonists

SAFETY OF DRUGS IN PREGNANCY (Contd...)

Class of medication	Relatively safe to use in pregnancy	Limited data or fetal risk appear minimal	Evidence of fetal risk	Significant fetal risk avoid in pregnancy
		Prazosin Procainamide Propranolol Quinidine Terazosin Timolol		
Cough and Cold agents			Dextromethorphan Phenylpro-panolamine Pseudoephedrine Amiloride Bumetanide Chlorthalidone Chlorthiazide Ethacrynic acid Furosemide Hydroclorothiazide Indapamide Metolazone Spironolactone Torsemide Triamterene	Guafensin
Gastrointestinal Misoprostol agents	Antacids Attapulgite Kaolin-pectin Loperamide Metoclopramide Psyllium	Bismuth subsalicylate Casanthranol Cisapride Dicyclomine Docusate H$_2$-receptor antagonists Lansoprazole Omeprazole Phenolphthalein Senna Simethicone Sucralfate		
Hormonal agent			Glucocorticoids (systemic) Progestins	Estrogens Oral contraceptive

SAFETY OF DRUGS IN PREGNANCY (Contd...)

Class of medication	Relatively safe to use in pregnancy	Limited data or fetal risk appear minimal	Evidence of fetal risk	Significant fetal risk avoid in pregnancy
Respiratory agents		Albuterol Beclomethasone (Inhalation) Ipratropium Metaproterenol Montelukast Nedocromil Pirbuterol Salmeterol Theophylline Triamcinolone (Inhalation) Zafirlukast	Zileuton	
Thyroid preparations		Levothyroxine	Potassium iodine Propylthiouracil	Methimazole
Miscellaneous	Ferrous sulphate Potassium chloride	Allopurinol	Azathioprine Carisoprodol	Isotretinion Cilosporine
Leflunomide Chlorzoxazone	Cyclosparine	Quinine Cyclobenzaprine Etanercept Flavoxate Oxybutynin	Modafinil Naratriptan Pentoxifylline Sumatriptan Rizatripan Zolmitriptan	Tamoxifen

EFFECTS OF LIPID LOWERING DRUGS ON LIPOPRTEIN LEVEL

		Lipoprotein level changes		
		LDL (mg%)	HDL Cholesterol (mg%)	Triglycerides Cholesterol (mg%)
1.	*Bile acid sequestrants*			
	(a) Cholestyramine	↓	↑ (slight)	None or ↑
	(b) Colestipol	↓	↑ (slight)	None or ↑
2.	*Nicotinic acid*	↓↓	↑↑	↓↓
3.	*Probucol*	↓	↓↓	None
4.	*Statins (HMG CoA reductase inhibitors)*			
	(a) Lovastatin	↓↓	↑	↓
	(b) Pravastatin	↓	↑	↓
	(c) Simvastatin	↓↓↓	↑	↓
5.	*Fibric acid derivatives*			
	(a) Gemfibrozil	↓	↑ to ↑↑	↓↓↓
	(b) Clofibrate	↓	↑	↓↓
	(c) Bezafibrate	↓	↑	↓↓↓
	(d) Fenofibrate	↓↓	↑	↓↓↓

↑ =5-15% change; ↑↑ = 15-30%; ↑↑↑ = > 30%

DIFFERENCES BETWEEN TUBOCURARINE AND DECAMETHONIUM

	Property	Tubocurarine	Decamethonium
1.	Action on the motor end plate	Block the action of Arch	Produces persistent depolarisation
2.	Initial excitation of the skeletal muscle	No excitation	Produces transient fasciculations
3.	Interaction with anticholinesterases	Antagonism	No antagonism
4.	Effect of prior administration of decamethonium	Additive	Antagonistic
5.	Effect of prior administration of decamethonium	Indifference or antagonism	Tachyphylaxis
6.	Effect on the avian skeletal	Flaccid paralysis	Spastic paralysis
7.	Effect on skeletal muscles of the cat	Paralyses respiratory musles (red) more than limb muscles (white)	Paralyses respiratory muscles less than limb muscles
8.	Effect of indirect tetanic stimulation during partial block	Poorly sustained contraction	Well sustained contraction
9.	Effect of application of catho-	Lessens paralysis	Intensifies paralysis
10.	Effect of application of anodal current to the end plate	Intensifies paralysis	Lessens paralysis

ANTIRETROVIRAL THERAPY

Drug	Indication	Dose	Common Side Effects	Monitoring
Zidovudine (AZT)	CD4 < 500 cells/ml.	500-600 mg orally daily in 3 divided doses	Anemia, neutropenia, nausea, malaise, headache, insomnia	Complete blood count and differential (every 3 months once stable).
Didanosine (dd)	CD4 < 500 cells.m*l and intolerant to AZT or with progestion of disease on AZT	125-300 mg orally twice a day (for pill formulation)	Peripheral neuropathy, pancreatitis, dry mouth	CBC and differential K+, amylase, triglycerides, monthly neurologic examination
Didocoxycytidine (ddC)		0.375-0.75 mg orally 3 times a day	Peripheral neuropathy, aphthous ulcers, transaminitis	Monthly neurologic examination, transaminases

SOME DRUGS KNOWN TO CAUSE LEUCOPENIA, AGRANULOCYTOSIS AND HEMOLYTIC REACTIONS

Drugs causing leucopenia and agranulocytosis	*Drugs causing hemolytic reactions*
Tranquillizers : Chlorpromazine and related drugs, Meprobamate	*Antibacterial agents :* Sulfonamides, Furazolidone, Nitrofurantoin, Chloramphenicol
Analgesics : Amidopyrine, Phenylbutazone, Oxyphenbutazone, analgin, Indomethacin	
Antibacterial agents : Chloramphenicol, Sulfonamides, Streptomycin, cotrimoxozole	*Antiprosy drugs (Sulfones) :* Diaminodiphenyl sulfone, Sulfoxone
Antithyroid drugs : Thiouracil, Propylthiouracil, Methimazole, Potassium perchlorate	*Antimalarials :* Primaquine, Pamaquine, Mepacrine, Quinine
Miscellaneous : Troxidone, Procainamide, Thiacetazone, Gold preparations, Imipramine.	*Miscellaneous drugs :* Acetanilid, Salicylates, Phenacetin, Naphthalene, Water soluble analogues of vitamin K Methyldopa.

COMPLICATIONS OF SERIOUS POISONING

Cardiogenic shock

　　direct action of drug on heart muscle

　　venous pooling in the lower limb

　　increased capillary permeability leading to reduced circulatory volume

Hypothermia

Convulsions

'Shock lung'—this complication is not often found, but should be considered

when there is inappropriate hyperventilation with non-respiratory alkalosis

THE ANTIDOTES OF MORPHINE, BARBITURATE, STRYCHNINE.

Drugs	Antidote
Morphine	Nalophine
Barbiturate	Analeptics, Bemegride
Bromide	Sodium chloride
Amphetamine	Haloperidol
Benzodiazepines	Flumazenil
Strychnine	Mephenesin.
Organophosphorus	Atropine, (oxine)
Heparin	Protomine sulphate
Dicoumarol	Vitamin K.
Heavy Metals	B.A.L. (for arsenic, mercury, gold).
Iron	Desferrioxamine
Lead, copper	Sod. calcium edetate, penicillamine
Curare	Neostigmine.
Cyanide	Nitrite followed by Thiosulphate
L.S.D.	Chlorpromazine.

DRUGS AND AGENTS TO BE AVOIDED IN LACTATION

Most drugs are excreted in the milk, but usually only in small amounts, which are neither beneficial not harmful to the baby. Exceptions are listed below :

1. Alcohol
2. Lithium
3. Antibiotics—Penicillins, Streptomycin & Nalidixic Acid, * Tetracyclines Sulphones
4. Metronidazole
5. Propranolol
6. Smoking
7. Steroids
8. Herbal Medicines—Coptis teeta
9. *Anticoagulants
10. Anticonvulsants—*Primidone
11. * Antithyroid Drugs—Thiouracil, Radioactive iodine.
12. Mothballs (Naphthalene)—Babies during their first 3 weeks must not use clothes exposed to naphthalene Moth-balls. Absorption of napthalene through the skin may precipitate haemolytic jaundice in G-6-PD deficient babies.
13. * Antitumour Drugs
14. Aspirin
15. Fluoride
16. Hypoglycaemic agents (oral)
17. Laxatives
18. Ergot preparations

* Do not breast feed

KEY TO FDA USE IN PREGNANCY RATINGS

The U.S. Food and Drug administrations use-in-pregnancy ratings system weighs the degree to which available information has ruled out risk to the fetus against the drugs potential benefit to the patient. The ratings and their interpretation, are as follows.

Category	Interrpretatation
A	Controlled studies show to risk. Adequate well controlled studies in pregnant women have failed to demonstrate a risk to the fetus in any trimester of pregnancy

B No evidence of risk in humans. Adequate well-controlled studies in pregnant women have not shown increased risk of fetal abnormalities despite adverse finding in animals or in the absence of adequate human studies, animal studies show no fetal risk. The chance of fetal harm is remote, but remains a possibility.

C Risk cannot be ruled out, Adequate, well controlled human studies are lacking and animal studies have shown a risk to the fetus or are lacking as well. There is a chance of fetal harm if the drug is administered during pregnancy but the potential benefits may outweigh the potential risk.

D Positive evidence of risk, Studies in humans, or investgational or post marketing data. have demonstrated fetal risk. Nevertheless, potential benefits from the use of the drug may outweigh the potential risk. For example, the drug may be acceptable if needed in a life threatening situation or serious disease for which safer drugs cannot be used or are ineffective.

X Contraindicated in pregnancy, Sudies in animals or humans, or investgational or post marketing reports have demonstrated positive evidence of fetal abnormalities or risk which clearly outweigh any possible benefit to the patient.

INFLUENCES ON DRUG METABOLISM BY PREGNANCY

1. ↑ GFR (clearance of digoxin, lithium).
2. ↑ Hepatic microsomal (P-450) enzyme activity
   — ↑ anticonvulsant metabolism.
3. ↑ Volume of distribution (eg. for cloxacillin).
4. ↑ Plasma protein binding (eg. aspirin, phenytoin).
5. ↑ Gastric emptying.

DRUGS TO BE AVOIDED IN G-6-P-D DEFICIENCY

Aspirin—Phenacetin—Actanilid—All sulpha derivatives—All Nitrofuran derivatives—Quinidine—Quinine—Primaquine—Pamaquine—Me pacrine—Arsenic derivative—PAS—BAL (Dimercaparol)—Diphen hydramine—Benemid—Chloramphenicol— Nitrites—Heavy doses of Vit. C—Chloroquine—Vit K—Sulphones (Dapsone).

RECOGNIZED TERATOGENS

1. *Warfarin* ('Koala bear' facies).
2. *Phenoytoin* (digital hypoplasia).
3. *Valproate (Na)* (spina bifida).
4. *Phenobarbitone* (cleft palate).
5. *Lithium* (Ebstein's anomaly).
6. *Thalidomide* (phocomelia).
7. *Ergometrine* (poland anomaly).
8. *Cytotoxics* especially methotrexate, alkylators.
9. *Steroid narmones*—
   Diethyl stiboesterol (DES) —vaginal Ca in adolescent female progeny.
   Androgens—cardiac/oesophageal defects.
10. *Alcohol* (acetaldehyde—metabolite foetal alcohol syndrome).
11. *Isotretinoin* (13-cis-retinoic acid), etretinate high dose, Vitamin D or Vitamin A.
12. *Radioisotopes* especially $I^{131.}$
13. *Live Vaccines*

CLINICAL MANIFESTATIONS OF ADVERSE REACTIONS TO DRUGS

I. **OCULAR MANIFESTATIONS**

   A. **Cataracts**
      Busulfan
      Chlorambucil
      Glucocorticoids
      Phenothiazines

   B. **Color vision alteration**
      Barbiturates
      Digitalis
      Methaqualone
      Streptomycin
      Sulfonamides
      Thiazides
      Troxidone

   C. **Corneal edema**
      Oral contraceptives

D. Corneal opacitles
Chloroquine
Indomethacin
Mepacrine
Vitamin D
E. Glaucoma
Mydriatics
Sympathomimetics
F. Optic neuritis
Aminosalicylic acid
Chloramphenicol
Clioquinol Ethambutol
Isoniazid
Penicillamine
Quinine
Streptomycin
G. Retinopathy
Chloroquine, Thioridazine

II. **EAR MANIFESTATIONS**
A. Deafnes
Aminoglycosides
Aspirin
Bleomycin
Chloroquine
Erythromycin
Ethacrynic acid
Furosemide
Mustine
Nortriptyline
Quinine
B. Vestibular disorders
Aminoglycosides
Mustine
Quinine

III. **MUSCULOSKELETAL MANIFESTATIONS**
A. Bone disorders
1. Osteoporosis :
Glucocorticoids
Heparin

   2. **Osteomalacia :**
     Aluminum hydroxide
     Anticonvulsants
     Glutethimide
 B. Myopathy or myalgia
    Amphotericin B
    Carbenoxolone
    Chloroquine
    Clofibrate
    Glucocorticoids
    Oral contraceptives
 C. Myositis
    Lovastatin

IV. PSYCHIATRIC MANIFESTATIONS
 A. Delirious or confusional
    Amantadine
    Aminophylline
    Anticholinergics
    Antidepressants
    Bromides
    Cimetidine
    Digitalis
    Glucocorticoids
    Isoniazid
    Levodopa
    Methyldopa
    Penicillins
    Phenothiazines
    Sedatives and hypnotics
 B. Depression
    Amphetamine withdrawal
    Beta blockers
    Centrally acting antihypertensives (reserpine, methyldopa, clonidine)
    Glucocorticoids
    Levodopa
    Phenothiazines
 C. Drowsines
    Antihistamines
    Anxiolytic drugs
    Clonidine
    Major tranquilizers
    Methyldopa
    Reserpine
    Tricyclic antidepressants

D. Hallucinatory states
Amantadine
Beta blockers
Levodopa
Meperidine
Narcotics
Pentazocine
Tricyclic antidepressants

E. Hypommania, mania, or excited reactions
Glucocorticoids
Levodpa
Meperidine
Narcotics
Pentazocine
Tricyclic antidepressants

F. Schizophrenic-like or paranoid reactions
Amphetamines
Bromides
Corticosteroids
Levodopa
Lysergic acid
Monoamine oxidase inhibitors
Sympathomimetics

V GASTROINTESTINAL MANIFESTATIONS

A. Cholestatic jaundice
Acetohexamide
Antabolic steroids
Androgens
Chlorpropamide
Erythromycin estolate
Gold salts
Methimazole
Nitrofurantoin
Oral contraceptives
Phenothiazines

B. Constipation or ileus
Aluminum hydroxide
Barium sulfate
Calcium carbonate
Ferrous sulfate
Ganglionic blockers
Ion exchange resins

Opiates
Phenothiazines
Tricyclic antidepressants
C. **Diarrhea or colitis**
Clindamycin
Colchicine
Digitalis
Guanethidine
Lactose excipients
Linomycin
Magnesium in antacids
Methyldopa
Purgatives
Reserpine
D. **Diffuse hepatocellular damage**
Acetaminiphen (paracetamol)
Allopurinol
Aminosalicylic acid
Aprindine
Dapsone
Erythromycin estolate
Ethionamide
Glyburide
Halothane
Isoniazid
Ketoconazole
Methimazole
Methotrexate
Methoxyflurane
Methyldopa
Monoamine oxidase inhibitors
Niacin
Nifedipine
Nitrofurantoin
Oxyphrenisatin
Phenytoin and other hydantoins
Propoxyphene
Propylthiouracil
Pyridium
Rifampin
Salicylates
Sodium valproate

Sulfonamides
Tetracyclines
Verapamil
Zidovudine (AZT)
Intestinal ulceraton
Solid KCl preparations

E. **Malabsorption**
Aminosalicylic acid
Antibiotics (broadspectrum)
Cholestyramine
Colchicine
Cytotoxics
Neomycin
Phenobarbital
Phenytoin
Primidone

F. **Nausea or vomiting**
Digitalis
Estrogens
Ferrous sulfate
Levodopa
Opiates
Potassium chloride
Tetracyclines
Theophylline

G. **Oral conditions**

1. *Dental discoloration :*
Tetracycline

2. *Drymouth :*
Anticholinergics
Clonidine
Levodopa
Methyldopa
Tricyclic antidepressants

3. *Gingival hyperplasia :*
Calcium antagonists
Cyclosporine
Phenytoin

H. **Salivary gland swelling :**
Bethanidine
Bretylium
Clonidine

Guanethidine
Iodides
Phenylbutazone

I. Taste disturbances :
Biguanides
Captropril
Griseofulvin
Lithium
Metronidazole
Penicillamine
Rifampin

J. Ulceration :
Aspirin
Cytotoxics
Gentian violet
Isoproterenol
Pancreatin

K. Pancreatitis
Azathioprine
Ethacrynic acid
Furosemide
Glucocorticoids
Opiates
Oral contraceptives
Sulfonamides
Thiazides

I. Peptic ulceration or hemorrhage
Arpirin
Ethacrynic acid
Glucocorticoids
NSAIDs
Reserpine (large doses)

VI. RENAL MANIFESTATIONS

A. Bladder dysfunction
Anticholinergics
Disopyramide
Monoamine oxidase inhibitors
Tricyclic antideprssants
Calculi
Acetazolamide
Vitamin D
Concentrating defect with polyuria (or oephrogenic diabetes insipidus)
Demeclocyline

Lithium
Methoxyflurane
Vitamin D
Hemorrhage cystitis
Cyclophosphamide
B. **Interstitial nephritis**
   Allopurinol
   Furosemide
   Penicillins esp. methicillin
   Sulfonamides
   Thiazides
   Nephropathies
   Due to analgesics (e.g. phenacetin)
C. **Nephrotic syndrome**
   Captopril
   Gold salts
   Penicillamine
   Phenindione
   Probenecid
D. **Obstructive uropathy**
   Extrarenal : methysergide
   Intrarenal : cytotoxics
   Renal dysfunction
   Cyclosporine
   NSAIDs
   Triamterene
E. **Renal tubular acidosis**
   Acetazolamide
   Amphotericin B
   Degraded tetracycline
F. **Tubular necrosis**
   Aminoglycosides
   Amphotericin B
   Cephaloridine
   Colistine
   Cyclosporin
   Methoxyflurane
   Polymyxins
   Radioiodinated contrast medium
   Sulfonamides
   Tetracyclines

VII. NEUROLOGIC MANIFESTATIONS

A. Exacerbation of myasthenia
Aminoglycosides
Polymyxins

B. Extrapyramidal effects
Butyrophenones, e.g. haloperidol
Levodopa
Methyldopa
Metoclopramide
Oral contraceptives
Phenothiazines
Reserpine
Tricyclic antidepressants

C. Headache
Bromides
Ergotamine (withdrawal)
Hydralazine
Indomethacin

D. Peripheral neuropathy
Aminodarone
Chloramphenicol
Chloraquine
Chlorpropamide
Cloquinol
Clofibrate
Demeclocycline
Disopyramide
Ethambutol
Ethionamide
Glutethimide
Hydralazine
Isoniazid
Methysergide
Metrinidazole
Mustine
Nalidixic acid
Nitrofurantoin
Perhexiline
Phenelzine
Phenytoin
Polymyxin, colistin
Procarbazine

Streptomycin
Tollbutamide
Tricyclic antidepressants
Vincristine

E. **Pseudotumor cerebri (or intracranial hypertension)**
Amiodarone
Glucocorticoids, mineralocorticoids
Hypervitaminosis A
Oral contraceptives
Tetracyclines

F. **Seizures**
Amphetamines
Analeptics
Imipramine
Isoniazid
Lidocaine
Lithium
Nilidixic acid
Penicillins
Phenothiazines
Physostigmine
Theophylline
Tricyclic antidepressants

G. **Stroke**
oral contraceptives

VIII. **CARDIOVASCULAR MANIFESTATIONS**
A. **Acute chest pain** (nonischemic)
Bleomycin

B. **Angina exacerbation**
Alpha blockers
Ergotamine
Excessive thyroxine
Hydralazine
Methysergide
Minoxidil
Nifedipine
Oxytocin
Propranolol withdrawal
Vasopressin

C. **Arrhythmias**
Adriamycin
Antiarhythmic drugs

Atropine
Anticholinesterases
Beta blockers
Daunomycin
Digitalis
Emetine
Guanethidine
Lithium
Papaverine
Phenothiazines, particularly thioridazine
Sympathomimetics
Thyroid hormone
Tricyclic antidepressants
Verapamil

D.   **AV block**
Clonidine
Methyldopa
Verapamil

E. **Cardiomyopathy**
Adriamycin
Daunorubicin
Emetine
Lithium
Phenothiazines
Sulfonamides
Sympathomimetics

F. **Fluid retention or congestive heart failure**
Carbenoxolone
Diazoxide
Estrogens
Indomethacin
Mannite
Minoxidil
Phenylbutazo
Propranolol
Steroids
Verapamil

G. **Hypotension**
Calcium channel blockers, eg. nifedipine
Citrated blood
Diuretics
Levodopa

Morphine
Nitroglycerin
Phenothiazines
Protamine
Quinidine

H. Hypertension
Analeptics
Angiotonsin
Clonidine withdrawal
Corticotropin
Cyclosporine
Glucocorticoids
Monoamine oxidase inhibitors with sysmpathomimetics
NSAIDs (some
Oral contraceptives
Plasma expanders
Sympathomimetics
Tricyclic antidepressants with sympathomimetics
Vasopressin

K Pericarditis
Emetine
Hydralazine
Methysergide
Procainamide

I Tachycardia
Adrenaline
Amyl nitrite
Atropine
Isoprenaline
Thyroxine (T4)

J Bradycardia
Digitalis
Methacholine
Neostigmine
Propranolol
Reserpine

L. Thromboembolism
Oral contraceptives

IX. **RESPIRATORY MANIFESTATIONS**
A. Airway obstruction
(bronchopasm, asthma)
Beta blockers
Cephalosporines

Cholinergic drugs

Nonsteroidal antiinflammatory drugs e.g. aspirin, indomethacin

Penicillins

Pentazocine

Streptomycin

Tartrazine (drugs with yellow dye)

B. Cough

Angiotensin-converting enzyme inhibitors

C. Nasal congestion

Decongestant abuse

Guanethidine

Isoproterenol

Oral contraceptives

D. Pulmonary edema

Contrast media

Heroin

Hydrochlorthiazide

Methadone

Propoxyphene

E. Pulmonary infiltrates

Amiodarone

Azothioprine

Bleomycin

Busulfan

Carmustine (BCNU)

Chlorambucil

Cyclophosphamide

Melphalan

Methotrexate

Methysergide

Mitomycin C

Nitrofurantoin

Procarbaxzine

Sulfonamides

F. Respiratory depression

Aminoglycosides

Hypnotics

Opiates

Polymyxins

Sedatives

Trimethaphan

X. MULTISYSTEM MANIFESTATION

A. Anaphylaxis
Cephalosporins
Demeclocycline
Dextran
Insulin
Iodinated drugs or contrast media
Iron dextran
Lidocaine
Penicillins
Procaine
Streptomycin
Sulfobromophthalein

B. Angioedema
Captopril
Enalapril
Lisinopril

C. Drug-induced lupus erythematosus
Acebutolol
Asparaginase
Barbiturates
Bleomycin
Cephalosporins
Hydralazine
Iodides
Isoniazid
Methyldopa
Phenolphthalcin
Phenytoin
Procainamide
Quinidine
Sulfonamides
Thiouracil

D. Fever
Aminosalicylic acid
Amphotericin B
Antihistamines
Novobiocin
Penicillins
Hyperpyrexia
Antipsychotics

E. **Serum sickness**
   Aspirin
   Penicillins
   Proptomycin
   Sulfonamides

XI. **DRUG INDUCED ENDOCRINE MANIFESTATIONS**

A. **Addisonian-like syndrome**
   Busulfan
   Ketoconazole

B. **Galactorrhea**
   Methyldopa
   Phenothiazines
   Reserpine
   Tricyclic antidepressants

C. **Gynecomastia**
   Calcium channel antagonists
   Digitalis
   Estrogens
   Ethionamide
   Griseofulvin
   Isoniazid
   Methyldopa
   Phenytoin
   Reserpine
   Spironolactone
   Testosterone

D. **Thyroid function tests, disorders of**
   Acetazolamide
   Amiodarone
   Bomsulfophthalcin
   Chlorpropamide
   Clofibrate
   Colestipol and nicotinic acid
   Dimeraprol
   Gold salts
   Iodides
   Lithium
   Oral contraceptives
   Phenindione
   Phenothiazines (long-term)
   Phenylbutazone
   Phenytoin

Sulfomnamides
Tolbutamide
F. **Vaginal carcinoma**
Diethy Istilbestrol (given to mother)
XII. **METABOLIC MANIFESTATIONS**
A. **Hyperbilirubinemia**
Novobiocin
Rifampin
B. **Hypercalcemia**
Antacids with absorbable alkali
Thiazides
Vitamin D
C. **Hyperglycemia**
Chlorthalidone
Diazoxide
Encainide
Ethacrynic acid
Furosemide
Glucocorticoids
Growth hormone
Oral contraceptive
Thiazides
D. **Hypoglycemia**
Insulin
Oral hypoglycemics
Quinine
E. **Hyperkalemia**
Angiotensin-converting enzyme inhibitors
Amiloride
Cytotoxics
Digitalis overdose
Heparin
Lithium
Potassium preparations including salt substitute
Potassium salts of drugs
Succinylcholine
Triamterene
F. **Hypokalemia**
Alkali-induced alkalosis
Amphotericin B
Carbenoxolone

Corticosteroids
Diuretics
Gentamicin
Insulin
Laxative abuse
Mineralocorticoids, some glucocorticoids
Osmotic diuretics
Tetracycline (degraded)
Theophylline
Vitamin B12

G. Hyperuricemia
Angiotensin II
Aspirin (low dose)
Chlorthalidone
Cortisone & cytolytics
Cytotoxics
Ethacrynic acid
Ethambutol
Fructose (IV)
Furosemide
Hyperalimentation
Thiazides

H. Hyponatremia
1. *Dilutional :*
     Carbamazepine
Chloropropamide
Cyclophosphamide
Diuretics
Octreotide
Vincristine
2. *Salt wasting :*
Diuretics
Enemas
Mannitol

1. Metabolic acidosis
Acetazolamide
Paraldehyde (degraded)
Phenformin
Salicylates
Spironolactone

J. Porphyria exacerbation
Barbiturates

Benegride
Chlordiazepoxide
Estrogens
Glutethimide
Griseofulvin
Meprobamate
Oral contraceptive
 Phenytoin
 Rifampin
 Sulfonamides
 Tolbutamide

Newer Questions

1. Which of the following drug is used in treatment of prophylaxis of Parkinsonism?
   A. Propranolol
   B. Sumitriptan
   C. Ergotamine
   D. Domperidone

2. Which is used in treatment of Toxoplasmosis?
   A. Artensunate
   B. Thiacetazone
   C. Ciprofloxacin
   D. Pyrimethamine

3. What is the reason of complicated penetration of some drugs through brain-blood barrier?
   A. High lipid solubility of a drug
   B. Meningitis
   C. Absence of pores in the brain capillary endothelium
   D. High endocytosis degree in a brain capillary

4. Tetrabenazine is used in:
   A. Multiple sclerosis
   B. Parkinsonism
   C. Huntington's chorea
   D. Resistant schizophrenia

5. Metabolic transformation (phase 1) is:
   A. Acetylation and methylation of substances
   B. Transformation of substances due to oxidation, reduction or hydrolysis
   C. Glucuronide formation
   D. Binding to plasma proteins

6. Mechanisms of transmembrane signaling are the following EXCEPT:
   A. Transmembrane receptors that bind and stimulate a protein tyrosine kinase

Ans. 1 A,   2 D,   3 C,   4 C,   5 B,   6 B

    B. Gene replacement by the introduction of a therapeutic gene to correct a genetic effect

    C. Ligand-gated ion channels that can be induced to open or close by binding a ligand

    D. Transmembrane receptor protein that stimulates a GTP-binding signal transducer protein (G-protein) which in turn generates an intracellular second messenger

7. Which of the following local anesthetics is a thiophene derivative?

    A. Procaine   B. Ultracaine

    C. Lidocaine   D. Mepivacaine

8. Which of the following statements concerning pantothinic acid functions are true:

    A. Active functional form is pyridoxal phosphate, which is an essential coenzyme for transamination and decarboxylation of amino acids in more than 50 different enzyme systems

    B. Essential constituent of coenzyme A, the important coenzyme for acyl transfer in the TCA cycle and de novo fatty acid synthesis

    C. An extremely important antioxidant, which protects cell membrane lipids from peroxidation by breaking the chain reaction of free radical formation to which polyunsaturated fatty acids are particularly vulnerable

    D. Coenzyme for several reactions involving CO_2 fixation into various compounds e.g. acetyl CoA to malonyl CoA (acetyl CoA carboxylase) – initial step in de novo fatty acid synthesis; propionyl CoA to methylmalonyl CoA (propionyl CoA carboxylase), pyruvate to oxaloacetate (pyruvate carboxylase)

9. These substances are vitamin-like compounds, EXCEPT:

    A. Choline

    B. Vitamin PP

    C. Vitamin U (methylmethioninesulfonil chloride)

    D. Orotate acid

10. This drug both inhibits an enzyme and indirectly enhances clearance of low density lipoproteins (LDL):

    A. Cholestyramine   B. Lovastatin

    C. Nicotinic acid   D. Probucol

Ans.   7 B,   8 D,   9 B,   10 B

11. Flushing caused by this drug can be reduced by taking it after meals and/or by pretreatment with aspirin:
    A. Lovastatin   B. Nicotinic acid
    C. Gemfibrozil   D. Probucol

12. Erenumab is a new drug in the treatment of:
    A. Multiple sclerosis   B. Migraine
    C. Parkinsonism   D. Alzheimer's disease

13. Ocrelizumab is a new drug approved in the treatment of:
    A. Refractory epilepsy   B. Cluster headache
    C. Progressive multiple sclerosis D. Japanese encephalitis

14. Hyperuricemia in gout is treated by except:
    A. Febuxostat   B. Fremanezumab
    C. Lesinurad   D. Sulfinpyrazone

15. Cryopyrin-associated periodic syndromes is treated by:
    A. Canakinumab   B. Eptinezumab
    C. Galcanezumab   D. Ocrelizumab

16. Indication for dihydrotachysterol administration is:
    A. Parathyroid hormone resistance
    B. Paget's disease
    C. Increased osteolysis
    D. Hypophosphatemia

17. Unwanted effect of plicamycin (formerly mithramycin) is:
    A. Diarrhea   B. Myelosuppression
    C. Nephrolithiasis   D. Metastatic calcifications

18. Following drugs are used in Swine flu except:
    A. Zanamivir   B. Oseltamivir
    C. Peramivir   D. Rimantadine

19. Lincozamides have the following unwanted effect:
    A. Nephrotoxicity
    B. Cancerogenity
    C. Pseudomembranous colitis
    D. Irritation of respiratory organs

20. All of the following antifungal drugs are antibiotics, EXCEPT:
    A. Amphotericin B   B. Nystatin
    C. Myconazol   D. Griseofulvin

Ans. 11 B, 12 B, 13 C, 14 B, 15 A, 16 D, 17 B,
        18 D, 19 C, 20 C

21. The drug belonging to gonadotropin-releasing hormone agonists is:
    A. Leuprolide   B. Tamoxifen
    C. Flutamide   D. Anastrozole
22. Zanamivir has the following side effects except:
    A. Dizziness   B. Breathing difficulties
    C. Mood changes   D. Seizures
23. Tick niclosamide mechanism of action:
    A. Increasing cell membrane permeability for calcium, resulting in paralysis, dislodgement and death of helminthes
    B. Blocking acetylcholine transmission at the myoneural junction and paralysis of helminthes
    C. Inhibiting oxidative phosphorylation in some species of helminthes
    D. Inhibiting microtubule synthesis in helminthes and irreversible impairment of glucose uptake
24. Blonanserin is useful in:
    A. Depression   B. Enuresis
    C. Tardive dyskinesia   D. Schizophrenia.
25. Tick the drug for cestodosis (tapeworm invasion) treatment:
    A. Piperazine   B. Praziquantel
    C. Pyrantel   D. Ivermectin
26. The drug, inhibiting uncoating of the viral RNA:
    A. Vidarabine   B. Acyclovir
    C. Rimantadine   D. Didanozine
27. The drug that can induce peripheral neuropathy and oral ulceration:
    A. Acyclovire   B. Zalcitabine
    C. Zidovudine   D. Saquinavir
28. Tick the drug that can induce nausea, diarrhea, abdominal pain and rhinitis:
    A. Acyclovire   B. Zalcitabine
    C. Zidovudine   D. Saquinavir
29. The mechanism of action of anticancer drugs belonging to plant alkaloids is:
    A. Inhibition of DNA-dependent RNA synthesis
    B. Cross-linking of DNA

Ans. 21 A,   22 D,   23 C,   24 D,   25 B,   26 C,   27 B,
          28 D,   29 C

   C. Mitotic arrest at a metaphase

   D. Nonselective inhibition of aromatases

30. Tick the drug belonging to aromatase inhibitors:

   A. Octreotide   B. Anastrozole

   C. Flutamide   D. Tamoxifen

31. Following are side-effects of Dutasteride used in BHP:

   A. Impotence

   B. Testicular pain and swelling

   C. Increased breast size

   D. Mania

32. Following are side effects of silodosin except:

   A. Nasal congestion   B. Retrograde ejaculation

   C. Diarrhoea   D. Seizures

33. Tick the drug of choice for herpes and cytomegalovirus infection treatment:

   A. Saquinavir   B. Interferon alfa

   C. Didanozine   D. Acyclovir

34. Tick the unwanted effects of fluoroquinolones:

   A. Hallucinations   B. Headache

   C. Hypertension   D. Immunotoxicity

35. Following are side effects of Bedaquiline used in MDR-TB except:

   A. Arrhythmias   B. Chest pain

   C. Hyperuricemia   D. Retinopathy

36. Amphotericin B has the following unwanted effects:

   A. Psychosis

   B. Anemia

   C. Hypertension, cardiac arrhythmia

   D. Bone marrow toxicity

37. Antibiotics altering permeability of cell membranes are:

   A. Glycopeptides   B. Polymyxins

   C. Tetracyclines   D. Cephalosporins

38. This drug is a desintoxicative plasma substitute:

   A. Polyglucinum

   B. Sodium chloridum isotonic for injections

   C. Haemodesum

   D. "Disolum", "Trisolum"

Ans.   **30 B,**   **31 D,**   **32 D,**   **33 D,**   **34 B,**   **35 D,**   **36 B,**
      37 B,   **38 C**

39. Spironolactone acts at this nephron site:
    A. Proximal convoluted tubule
    B. Ascending thick limb of the loop of Henle
    C. Distal convoluted tubule
    D. Collecting duct

40. Indications for etidronate administration are the following, EXEPT:
    A. Paget's disease   B. Osteoporosis
    C. Hypophosphatemia   D. Hypercalcemia

41. Bemegride:
    A. Stimulates the medullar respiratory center (central effect)
    B. Stimulates hemoreceptors of carotid sinus zone (reflector action)
    C. Is a mixed agent (both central and reflector effects)
    D. Is a spinal analeptic

42. Sydnocarb (a CNS Psychostimulant) causes:
    A. Decreased sense of fatigue, it facilitates the professional work and fights somnolence
    B. The feeling of prosperity, relaxation and euphoria
    C. Influx of physical and mental forces, locomotive and speech excitation
    D. Peripheral sympathomimetic action

43. Folowing are true about newer antidepressant, Vortioxetine except:
    A. 5HT1A agonist   B. 5HT-1B partial antagonism
    C. 5HT – 1D antagonism   C. 5HT-7 antagonism

44. Tolcapone, a antiparkinsonian drug, is a:
    A. Dopamine agonist   B. MAO-B inhibitor
    C. COMT inhibitor   D. Anticholinergic drug

45. Rasagiline, an antiparkinsonian drug has following side effects except:
    A. Joint pain   B. Dizziness
    C. Pancreatitis   D. Hallucinations

46. A general tone-increasing drug, which is an agent of animal origin?
    A. Pantocrin   B. Amphetamine
    C. Sydnocarb   D. Camphor

47. Following are side effects of Alogliptin, a newer antidiabetic drug, except:

Ans. 39 D,   40 C,   41 A,   42 A,   43 B,   44 C,   45 C,
      46 A,   47 A

A. Weight gain   B. Mild hypoglycemia
C. Joint pain   D. Risk of heart failure

48. Flumazenil is used for following except:
   A. To reverse the CNS depressant effects of hypnotic benzo-diazepines overdose
   B. To hasten recovery following use of hypnotic benzodiazepines in anesthetic and diagnostic procedure
   C. To reverse benzodiazepine-induced respiratory depression
   D. To treat mixed overdose or benzodiazepine tolerance

49. Which of the following benzodiazepines is preferred for elderly patients?
   A. Clorazepate   B. Clordiazepoxide
   C. Triazolam   D. Prazepam

50. Following drugs may induce stuttering except:
   A. Theophylline   B. Fluoxetine
   C. Gabapentin   D. Phenytoin

51. Limitation of buspirone is:
   A. A low therapeutic index
   B. An extremely slow onset of action
   C. A high potential of development of physical dependence
   D. Impairment of mentation or motor functions during working hours

52. Indicate the following neuromuscular blocker, which would be contraindicated in patients with renal failure:
   A. Pipecuronium   B. Succinylcholine
   C. Atracurium   D. Rapacuronium

53. The neuromuscular blocker, which causes tachycardia:
   A. Tubocurarine   B. Atracurium
   C. Pancuronium   D. Succinylcholine

54. A ganglion-blocking drug, which can be taken orally for the treatment of hypertension?
   A. Mecamylamine   B. Scopolamine
   C. Trimethaphane   D. Vecocuronium

55. M3 receptor subtype is located:
   A. In the myocardium
   B. In sympathetic postganglionic neurons

Ans. 48 D,   49 C,   50 D,   51 B,   52 A,   53 C,   54 A,   55 C

    C. On effector cell membranes of glandular and smooth muscle
       cells

    D. On the motor end plates

56. Isofluorophate increases all of the following effects except:
    A. Lacrimation   B. Bronchodilation
    C. Muscle twitching   D. Salivation

57. Ionizable group is responsible for:
    A. The potency and the toxicity
    B. The duration of action
    C. The ability to diffuse to the site of action
    D. All of the above

58. Drugs which can cause pancreatitis include following except:
    A. Valproic acid   B. Tetracycline
    C. Thiazide   D. Anastrozole

59. Following are newer antiepileptic drugs except:
    A. Felbamate   B. Topiramate
    C. Linagliptin   D. Fosphenytoin

60. Prasugrel, a newer antiplatelet drug, has following side effects
    except:
    A. A severe allergic reaction   B. Headache
    C. Nausea   D. Epistaxis

Ans.   56 B,   57 C,   58 D,   59 C,   60 A